BORN TO BE BRAD

BORN TO BE BRAD

MY LIFE AND STYLE, SO FAR

Brad Goreski

WITH MICKEY RAPKIN

*it*books

AN IMPRINT OF HARPERCOLLINS PUBLISHERS

BORN TO BE BRAD. Copyright © 2012 by Brad Goreski. All rights reserved.
Printed in the United States of America. No part of this book may be used or
reproduced in any manner whatsoever without written permission except in the case
of brief quotations embodied in critical articles and reviews. For information address
HarperCollins Publishers, 10 East 53rd Street, New York, NY 10022.

HarperCollins books may be purchased for educational, business, or sales
promotional use. For information please write: Special Markets Department,
HarperCollins Publishers, 10 East 53rd Street, New York, NY 10022.

FIRST EDITION

Designed by Renato Stanisic

Library of Congress Cataloging-in-Publication Data has been applied for.

ISBN 978-0-06-212537-8

12 13 14 15 16   ov/oG   10 9 8 7 6 5 4 3 2 1

*To my mom, my sister, my grandma Ruby, and all of the other
amazing women who have inspired me along the way*

And to the man who continues to inspire me, my boyfriend, Gary Janetti

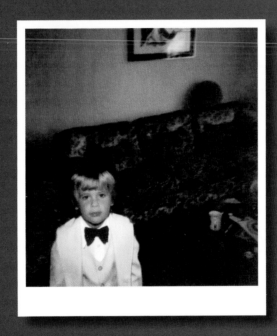

CONTENTS

Prologue:
Playing dress-up isn't
just for kids.

I WAS FIVE YEARS old, and I was already on trend. For the first day of kindergarten, I was dressed in corduroy pants, a pair of sneakers, and a snug little jacket. I was also wearing nail polish. Why? Because I idolized my mother. She looked like a fashion plate to me, and she never left the house without nail polish. And so, on the first day of school, neither did I. That's what ladies do.

The classroom was full of books and crayons, and there were different play stations set up for us kids, which were clearly divided along gender lines. On the left were the trucks and G.I. Joes for the boys, and on the right a pretend kitchenette and some dolls for the girls. You can probably guess which side of the room I gravitated toward.

My teacher was Mrs. Chandler, and she was the most fashionable woman I had ever seen. She was dressed in an A-line skirt, with a proper cardigan and a poet blouse with a perfect bow tied at the top. She was rather elegant for a schoolteacher, with her jet-black hair and fancy French beret. Oh, and the costume jewelry! And the sensible heels! I didn't have a vocabulary for these things back then but I knew how they made me feel: like something more was possible.

My love for dressing people started right there, the same way it did for most girls: with Barbie. As a kid in Port Perry, Ontario (population 9,500), I would dress that iconic plastic blonde in the best gowns, styling her hair in an updo to accentuate her long neck. I didn't know what a stylist was. I didn't know it was an actual job. But I knew how it felt to play dress-up. I knew that fashion could be a transformative experience, for Barbie and for me. I knew that when the kids on the playground called me names, I could escape in the pages of fashion magazines. I discovered that even normal clothing could feel like a costume. You could be someone else. And dress-up was magic.

My strongest memory from kindergarten isn't learning the letters of the alphabet but rather learning to recognize Mrs. Chandler's different looks. I saw something special in her. And I know she saw something special in me, too. At an early parent-teacher meeting, I found out years later, she sat down with my sometimes-confused mother to say, "Don't ever dampen his spirit. He'll be fine." My mom knew I was different. But I think she took comfort in having confirmation from someone else.

I have been blessed to have women like Mrs. Chandler in my life at every turn, and always when I needed them most. Powerful, smart, beautiful women who never discouraged me from playing with Barbie dolls, who never told me to tone down my voice or my mannerisms, who never wanted me to be anything but myself. Which was fairly revolutionary

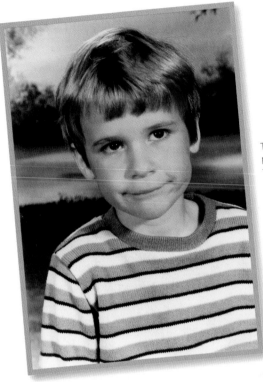

This is my kindergarten photo, and a fashion transition look from the seventies to the eighties.

for a reserved town in the early eighties. Mrs. Chandler saw me playing with dolls but didn't feel the need to pull me away or call my parents down to the school. Because she knew there was nothing wrong with me. She saw a spark, and rather than blow it out, she fanned the flames (so to speak), even though she probably knew the road wouldn't be easy. That's what all of these women in my life have done: my grandma Ruby, my mom, my sister, my bosses at *Vogue,* my friends in fashion. They protected me from bullies, from boyfriends, from a sometimes-cruel world, and prepared me for what was next. It is to these women that I owe everything.

And it has been quite a ride. While it is not very Canadian to champion yourself, I am proud of how far I've come—from my days as a fat kid in Port Perry and my struggles as a young adult who always felt on the outside looking in, someone who knew where the party was and knew exactly how far he was from it, to the front row at New York Fashion Week. On September 17, 2010, I was on the cover of the Styles section of the Sunday *New York Times,* dressed in a full Lanvin look. The piece recounted how I was front row at the Simon Spurr show and backstage at Michael Bastian. Joe Zee, the creative director of *Elle* magazine, was interviewed, describing me as "a style icon for this entire new generation of young, cool, preppy, dapper guys." Cameron Diaz told the story of an

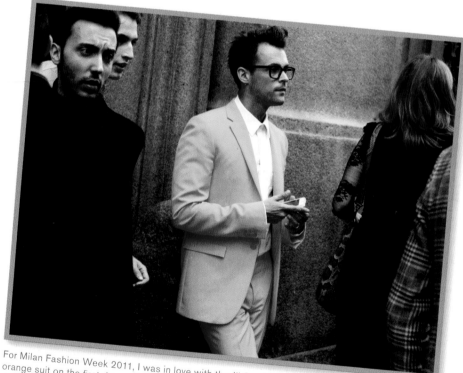

For Milan Fashion Week 2011, I was in love with the Jil Sander men's collection. I wore this orange suit on the first day, and it caused quite a storm. People were following me around all day taking my picture.

Oscar emergency, saying of that high-pressure afternoon, "Brad was able to help me concoct a heel pad out of a toe pad literally as I was running to the car." The *Times* piece ended with my crossing the street. As a taxi splashed me, I laughed, "That was my *Sex and the City* moment."

Against all odds, I am living a dream. After college, I worked as a fashion assistant at *Vogue* magazine's West Coast office, helping out on a dozen high-concept, high-end photo shoots with world-class photographers like Mario Testino. Me? The kid with buckteeth who used to tap-dance in talent shows? The kid who hung a commemorative Marilyn Monroe dinner plate on his bedroom wall? Believe me, I was as surprised as anyone to find myself there, and then on television, in your living room every week, frantically looking for the perfect dress for an A-list celeb. Especially since I'd made some serious fashion faux pas myself over the years. Like that terrible Von Dutch phase I went through when I first moved to L.A., when I thought it was OK to wear a pair of oversize Dior shield sunglasses with novelty T-shirts and cargo shorts. I had blond highlights, and my hair was all nappy with split ends.

There were other fashion mistakes, believe me. Like the time I went on a cruise with my boyfriend, and I wore Tom Ford for Gucci raw denim, flared Western jeans with a Gucci logo belt, pointy suede Dolce & Gabbana boots, a white shirt, and a Gucci handkerchief around my neck. I had a Sears-catalog blond haircut and I looked like Ellen DeGeneres dressed as a cowgirl.

And yet my story has all the elements of a fashion fairy tale—with trips overseas and celebrity clients and the chance to work with some of the most beautiful clothing in the world. But what's less known is that, at its heart, mine is also a survival story—of too much partying, which I used to dull the pain of a sometimes difficult childhood. In my early twenties, I came to a fork in the road and I had to make a choice: Would I continue to abuse myself, or would I listen to the voice of those women in my life, the ones who told me I could be so much more?

This was harder than it may seem. People from Port Perry don't just pack up a U-Haul and leave town for New York. Most of the people stay and take over the family business. And for them that's enough. For them, that works. As a kid, I may have been in the basement with my mother adding plaid borders to the bottoms of my jeans and gluing sequins on everything in reach, but no one had any idea I'd make a career of this. That you could even *make* a career of this. Even I didn't see it. (I wanted to be a plastic surgeon, actually.) But reading fashion magazines, taping the Tony Awards off the television—it was a window to another world, and it made me realize there was something more out there for me. That if I listened to that same voice that told me Barbie should wear her hair off her face, I'd make something happen for myself. I didn't always know where I was going. That's part of the reason I loved fashion. I knew you could play dress-up and be whatever it is you wanted to be that day. And throughout my life, I tried on different personalities, different careers, trying to listen to my voice and see where I was heading. You don't need to be locked into one look or one strict personality; that much I know.

I have more to offer in this book than advice on how to get the perfect wardrobe, though there will be plenty of that, too. (Five must-have accessories every woman should own: a great closed-toe pump, a large day bag, a vintage clutch, an amazing pair of sunglasses, and a cocktail ring.) What I am offering, through my story, is proof that you can be your best self, whoever that may be. That you can change your life. That if you listen to the voice in your heart, you will succeed.

Look, I know: Age thirty-three might be a little early to be writing a memoir. I get it. I'm not Jane Fonda. (I wish.) The stories here may not be entirely unique. An overweight gay kid pursuing musical theater and obsessed with fashion? Shocker! But it is what we do with the information in front of us that is vital. How do you get from point A to point B when the steps in between seem like such a mystery?

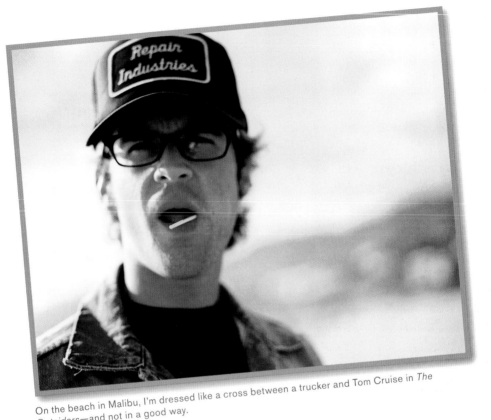

On the beach in Malibu, I'm dressed like a cross between a trucker and Tom Cruise in *The Outsiders*—and not in a good way.

What I know is: I got this far. I am a stylist working with clients whose talent I respect. I am ten years sober as of May 3, 2011. This was not some rocket to stardom. A lot was put in my way. My resources were limited. I didn't have connections. I wasn't born into this world. I just told anyone who would listen that I wanted to work in fashion. That I had a point of view. And when an opportunity presented itself, I did the work. I rolled up my sleeves and dug in my heels. It took sacrifices. There were times I wanted to quit. There were times where I got so close to the party that I could taste the mini-burgers, but even then it all felt like too much.

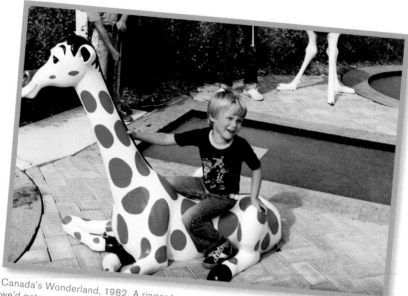

Canada's Wonderland, 1982. A ringer tee and jeans? I still wear this look. Incidentally, we'd get season passes to the amusement park. But my mom never wanted me to go alone. She was convinced that I'd die on a roller coaster or that someone would offer me drugs in the bathroom stalls.

My sobriety has a lot to do with pushing me forward. I didn't believe that I got sober to be miserable.

What I want to say is: Thank God I didn't change. Thank God I didn't compromise who I was, because I would not be here today. Being yourself comes with a price. I know that. It comes with a lot of adversity. You will run into people who want to bring you down. Especially when you become successful. I am telling my story here—in bold detail—because I want you to know that you don't have to change. That there is a world out there just waiting for you, exactly as you are.

What I'm offering is part style guide, part inspirational story about allowing yourself to fail, about listening to your heart and seeing where it leads you. That's the message of this book. Ignore the bullies, whether they're from the playground or the office, and find out where your passion lives. Look around and engage and take notes. And when you're ready, make it happen. This story is divided into three distinct sections: "Listen," "Look," "Leap."

I will take you to the red carpet at the Oscars, to photo shoots in far-flung locations, to the European runway shows, and to my childhood bedroom, where you'll find the purple faux-fur jacket I wore to the prom still hanging in the closet. This is the inspirational story of a kid who didn't fit in. A kid who left a small town in

> "Ignore the bullies, whether they're from the playground or the office, and find out where your passion lives."

Canada and somehow made his way to the offices of *Vogue* magazine and then into your living room. Get ready. Life hasn't been all bow ties and glasses. It's been glamorous but also rough at times.

LISTEN

1

The bullies may be loud. But your heart can beat louder.

I WAS TWELVE YEARS old when I started reading *Vogue*. Even before that I was always watching *Fashion Television*, a Canadian TV show that aired Sunday nights after the local news and was hosted by Jeanne Beker. She was Canada's answer to Elsa Klensch (still is) and I was obsessed with her. I can still hear the theme song in my head (*"I have an obsession . . ."*). Ask any Canadian why they got into fashion and Jeanne Beker's name will come up. She reported from the fashion shows in Milan and New York with such intensity—as if she was a war correspondent reporting from the front lines. Except these were the front lines of fashion. Needless to say, as a kid

living for *Fashion Television* and fighting with his sister over the remote
control—so he could watch *The Sound of Music* again—I wasn't a big hit
with the other Canadian boys in my school. I didn't care. I was sitting
at the kitchen table flipping through junk mail catalogs addressed to my
mom and picking out outfits for her. When she was getting ready to go out
for the night with my father, I'd go into her closet and grab a pair of denim
stirrup pants and a mid-thigh-length T-shirt for her to wear. I'd pester her:
"Don't you have a bracelet for that outfit?" In department stores, I'd walk
by the women's shoe department and shriek, "Mommy, those shoes!"

It's important to visualize where we are: I grew up in Port Perry, a
small eighteenth-century town on the banks of Lake Scugog in Ontario.
Don't ask me what "Scugog" means. I don't know the answer. What I do
know is that the buildings in town had gingerbread trim, a faux country
aesthetic that went nicely with the penny loafers and starched oxford
shirts my mom dressed me in
as a kid. My hometown looked
like the setting for a movie
with Meredith Baxter Birney,
and my childhood was about

> **"My childhood was about trying to
> fit a round kid in a square town."**

trying to fit a round kid in a square town. *Fashion Television* was like some
dispatch from a foreign planet. A place where I belonged. And for the first
of many times in my life, I became aware that there was a party going on
somewhere, but I was hopelessly on the outside looking in.

I dreamed of being an adult, of being thirty years old, because that
meant I would be my glamorous self somewhere far away. It's funny to
imagine an eight-year-old child starting every sentence with the phrase,
"When I turn thirty . . ." But I did, because that was my magic age. I
didn't know where I'd be or what I'd be doing. But I knew there wouldn't
be gingerbread houses. I was dreaming of another world. Or *Another
World*. I'd watch soap operas after school, and I was obsessed with Linda
Dano, who played Felicia Gallant. Felicia owned the chic store in Bay City,

and she loved herself a hat and a knee-length coat and a beaded smock, sometimes all at once. She was sophisticated, and I bought into the idea that hers was a very sophisticated boutique despite the cardboard backdrop. Soap operas are full of smoke and mirrors and glitter, but this became my idea of glamour.

My childhood misadventures didn't end with catalogs or soap operas. Sometimes, when my mother left the house, I'd go into her closet and dig out the veil she wore to my christening. I'd twirl around, looking at myself in the mirror and thinking for the first time, "I'm pretty." As you can imagine, my dad—a manager of a medical lab in nearby Oshawa— wasn't exactly thrilled. But he didn't pull away. He didn't shame me. In fact, the opposite happened. In the third grade, when the boys at school were dressing like their favorite hockey players for Halloween, I dressed up like Madonna. I made the costume myself, using one of Barbie's lace nighties as a glove. Sometimes you have to get creative and make things happen, even as a third grader, to get a message across. I wore a T-shirt cinched at the waist like a dress, and a pair of my mom's heels, and, yes, lipstick. I'm sure my dad would have preferred it if I'd chosen another costume, like a fireman or a police officer. We lived in a subdivision called Apple Valley, and none of the other little boys there were wearing lipstick. But there was a lot of love in my dad's heart. He put on a brave face, took my lace-gloved hand in his own, and dragged me around the neighborhood ringing doorbells.

It's no surprise that when I think of my childhood, I see it in terms of shifting sartorial inspirations. I made bold choices. And not all of them good choices. A look back:

Age eleven: To my communion, I wore a white suit with a spread-collar, pastel-colored Hawaiian shirt. I had blond hair and I was going for a Don Johnson, *Miami Vice* moment. You can judge how successful this was for yourself by looking at this photo. But I considered myself to be the best-dressed in the Catholic church, by far.

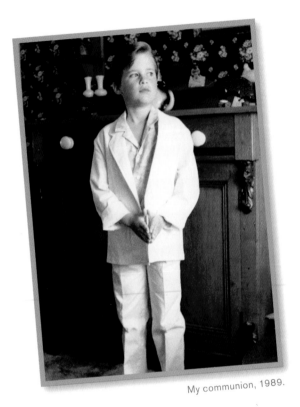

My communion, 1989.

Age twelve: As a family, we went to see the Jacksons' Victory Tour, and I was tenth-row center for Michael's performance of "Beat It." Thanks to some super-awesome special effect I'll never quite understand—I like to think it was magic—Michael disappeared into thin air. My mind disappeared, too, when I spotted the Victory Tour T-shirt with baby-blue sleeves and an iron-on of Tito and Jermaine for sale. My parents bought this T-shirt for me, and I wore it to school for weeks, pairing it with black jogging pants that had zippers down the sides; when you opened the zippers neon yellow fabric peeked through for a pop of color. As if that wasn't enough *look,* I tied a comic-book-print scarf asymmetrically around my waist. In case there's any question out there, this was a big fashion don't.

Age thirteen: I discovered Le Château, a store specializing in bold fashions in flammable fabrics. It was just another mall chain, but to me it felt like some terribly important Parisian boutique. The executives at Le Château's headquarters I'm sure never guessed it, but this place was epic for a young gay kid looking for more than a pair of jeans and a T-shirt. It was the only store at the mall with anything that appealed to us. At thirteen, I bought a charcoal-gray Le Château shirt with a velvet number 5 on the front. Now, I know what you're thinking. We've all had that moment: You're out shopping one afternoon and you fall in love with a piece of clothing but think, Where am I going to wear a charcoal shirt with a velvet number 5 on the front? Well, in this case, *everywhere*. To drama club practice with a pair of jeans. To school with black velvet jean-style trousers.

Looking in the mirror back then I thought I looked super-cool, but the kids at school didn't see it that way. Actually, they thought I looked like a

What Goes Around Comes Around

NEVER THROW ANYTHING AWAY. IT'S ALWAYS COMING BACK.

When J.Crew and Jil Sander both started selling bright colors for Spring/Summer 2011, I realized that old maxim really is true: What goes around comes around. Everything old is new again. This is why we have basements and storage units and deep closets; never throw anything away. Bass penny loafers? I stopped wearing them in high school when grunge came in, but they had a massive resurgence with the preppy movement in the mid-2000s. Speaking of grunge, as I write this, flannels and parkas are back in for a nineties moment. For women, denim jumpsuits and denim-on-denim (the Canadian tuxedo) are both socially acceptable again. If there's one item from my past that I wish I'd saved, it's an amazing *Les Misérables* T-shirt.

huge fag. The F-word? Yeah, a bully first called me that in the third grade. That was only the beginning.

My sister, Mandy, refers to our childhood home as the Kennedy Compound. And it had an air of Hyannis Port about it. My grandfather Phillip bought a large tract of land on Lake Scugog and sold the subdivisions off to the family piece by piece. My parents and my sister and I lived in a house on Percy Crescent, with aunts and uncles and cousins on all sides. We could see my grandparents' house from our backyard.

Everyone in town knew the Goreskis, because our grandfather Phillip owned the local resort, Goreski's Lakeside Recreation, a trailer park in the best sense of the word. He started the business in 1963, and it grew to include eight hundred trailer sites plus boat slips and a marina, two swimming pools, and a miniature golf course. Families came annually for the entire summer. What were the people like? It wasn't the chicest crowd. The boys wore Metallica T-shirts and jeans and bad high-tops, which at the time I found mildly offensive (however, in later years it would be a look I'd try to copy; things always come around). The young girls were scantily clad. And there I was in my polo shirt, cuffed jeans, and penny loafers, my hair always done. I stood out even at my family's resort. As kids, my sister, Mandy, and I worked at Goreski's Lakeside. She eventually

Burning question: Brad, please settle this once and for all. Is it OK to wear white after Labor Day?

This is one of those questions that persists over the ages. I have to say, I couldn't care less. And neither could designers. I was in YSL and saw a gorgeous white cashmere coat. It's called *winter white* for a reason. Because you're supposed to wear it in the winter.

ran the kitchen (as a teenager!), cooking up eggs, hamburgers, and fish-and-chips while I rang up the customers out front. For some people, working in a greasy take-out diner would be the worst summer job. But as an overweight kid, this was Candy Land—literally. I had access to all of the candy and ice cream I could eat. That is, until my uncle Ron fired me. I couldn't blame him. Cadbury was running a contest, and I opened every single Cadbury caramel looking for the golden ticket. I was Canada's answer to Veruca Salt. I want an Oompa-Loompa now, Daddy.

My sister had her own sense of style. Sometimes she dressed like a businessman, in a button-up and trousers. Other times she wore jeans and blazers. (She dresses the same way now.) Getting her to wear a dress and makeup became my mission in my youth. I succeeded once or twice; however, it never really took. I ended up wearing more dresses and makeup than she ever did. But she was my protector, and I am forever grateful to her. In grade five, for Halloween I dressed as the Wicked Witch of the West, which didn't go over so well. I wore a black turtleneck, with a red sequined spiderweb on the front of it and a glittery spider stuck to the web. The skirt was this shredded mess of black and red fabric, and then I had a long cape on a black sequined headband. It was a riff, not an exact replica. Three boys from my class cornered me in the hallway and threatened to beat me up. Thankfully, a teacher came by and broke it up before they could land a punch. But my sister really let them know what was up. Out on the playground later that day, she tracked down those three boys and said, "If you're planning on hurting anyone, you'll have to answer to me first." And then she pounded the crap out of them.

I was not the little boy from all of those television sitcoms—the one who tells his sister to back off, the one who insists he can fight his own battles. I just accepted that this was my lot in life. And I could no more change these boys than change who I was. Mandy was another of those superhero women in my life watching over me. Though I certainly didn't make it easy for her. When she won the school's citizenship award and

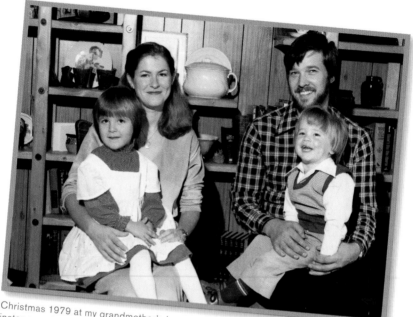

Christmas 1979 at my grandmother's house. This is one of the few documented instances of my sister, Mandy, wearing a dress.

she went up to receive the trophy, I stood up in front of all five hundred students and shouted with a lisp, "That's my *sister*!" That was me. I was *dramatic*. I was the performer in the family. At the time, I was taking dance lessons. And when Grandpa Phillip had family over to the house, he'd parade me around the dining room saying, "Bradley, I'll pay you five bucks to dance for me." I happily took the five dollars, though I would have done it for free.

> "That was me. I was *dramatic*. I was the performer in the family."

My grandfather Harry, meanwhile, was a pharmacist and my mother worked in his office, putting on her starched white uniform every day.

Sometimes I went to the pharmacy after school, sitting in the back, playing on the calculator and eating chocolate bars while waiting for my mom—anything to avoid riding on the school bus with the other kids. Though I could stomach the bus ride if it meant getting off at our grandma Ruby's house. My sister and I would sometimes take the bus to her house, skipping down the hill, the smell from her kitchen getting stronger the closer we got. When I look back, I like to think I looked like Laura Ingalls in the opening credits to *Little House on the Prairie* as I ran down that hill, though maybe I looked more like Julie Andrews in *The Sound of Music*. But in reality, I was wearing a full snowsuit and moon boots, and I'd throw my head back and shout, "She's making roast beef and steamed apple pudding!" Like most chubby kids, I had an excellent sense of smell. I was a cartoon character, Preppy Le Pew, floating on air to the kitchen.

When we arrived, Ruby would be sitting in her rocking chair or standing in front of the kitchen stove beyond the saloon doors. Their house was a fifteen-hundred-square-foot cottage, with a pump organ where I'd sit waiting for a snack, banging on the pedals. "Bradley, stop playing that goddamn organ!" Grandma Ruby would shout out from the kitchen. That's how she spoke. She was a buxom woman, and vocal. We'd go shopping, and when my mother refused to buy me something I'd sometimes cry. Ruby would shout out, "Bradley, *I'll* give you something to cry about!"

In a sometimes-rocky childhood, Ruby was the constant. When I was in kindergarten, our parents briefly separated. Though they soon reconciled, that threat of instability loomed over our house forever. Whenever our parents would have a big disagreement, my sister and I would ask each other, "Do you think they'll get divorced?" But Ruby never wavered. She taught me to appreciate glamour. She had her hair done once a week, a permanent, of course. She was old-school in her charms. She preferred sensible shoes and cotton shirts with a cardigan over them, and a locket around her neck every day—work clothing, because what she did around

Dessert Oasis

GRANDMA RUBY'S RECIPE FOR FRENCH SILK PIE

TO MAKE THE FILLING

1 cup sugar
¾ cup butter, cut up
3 squares of unsweetened chocolate, melted and heated through
1½ teaspoons vanilla
3 eggs
1 pie shell, baked and cooled (recipe below)
Cool Whip for the top (optional)

Using a steel-blade processor, combine sugar and butter until very smooth and light, stopping to scrape down the sides of the bowl. Leave the processor running, and add chocolate and vanilla through the feed tube. Add eggs one at a time through the tube and process until the mixture is smooth. Turn into cooled pie shell and chill several hours or overnight.

TO MAKE THE PIE SHELL

5 cups flour
2 tablespoons sugar
1 teaspoon salt
1 pound lard (Tenderflake preferably)
1 egg
Water

Preheat the oven to 350˚F. Mix flour, sugar, and salt together, then cut in lard. Beat egg slightly in measuring cup, then add water to measure 1 cup of liquid. Mix together and roll into a 9-inch pie pan. Bake for 30 to 35 minutes.

the house was work. She was famous for baking. At Christmas, people couldn't wait for her to drop off her famous cookie trays. But she was modern, too, especially in her unfailing acceptance of me. She took me to auction sales. She taught me how to act around the dinner table and how to act around adults. She had a toy room in her house with antique toys, model planes hanging from the ceiling and dolls everywhere, and we could play with them. She never criticized me for playing with dolls or Barbie, whom I loved because she always had somewhere to go. She always had a big date at night or an event. She barely had any day looks because she didn't work. Barbie was all about night looks, and she existed to be glamorous. What is the impact of having your grandmother sit you down, put on a movie musical, and tell you anything is possible? I'm here to tell you it's immeasurable.

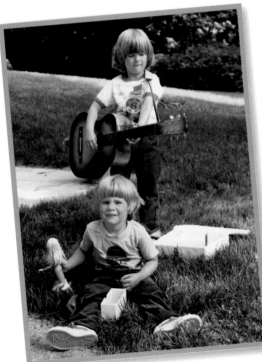

My sister never took a guitar lesson, but she certainly loved to wear the damn thing around her neck. I have my own favorite accessory here: a Barbie doll. She's naked because she's changing outfits.

Ruby's most important contribution might have been Marilyn Monroe. Our local supermarket, the Value Mart, was selling black-and-white photographs of Hollywood stars like Humphrey Bogart and the Three Stooges. But one day, there she was. I was twelve years old and holding this photo of her in a silver plastic frame with this border that was supposed to look like the lights of a dressing room mirror. I became obsessed with Marilyn—with her look, with her skin—yet I hadn't seen any of her movies. So Ruby plopped me down in front of the television, put on *Gentlemen Prefer Blondes,* and taught me to appreciate a good movie musical. All I needed to see was Marilyn in the pink dress singing "Diamonds Are a Girl's Best Friend." From then on, I was obsessed with blondes. When my aunt Kim got married, I refused to dance with anyone who didn't have doll-colored hair.

Which sort of explains what happened next. In grade eight, my English teacher asked everyone in the class to prepare a presentation on someone we admired. You can guess who I chose. By now, photos of the late icon covered my bedroom walls. I had a Marilyn Monroe commemorative plate from the Franklin Mint hanging by my bed. Of course I couldn't do just any presentation. I wanted to put on something as dramatic as, and as worthy of, her life. And so I produced a video presentation, which my sister and I shot on my uncle's video camera—the kind that was like a VCR with a lens attached to it. It was a two-day shoot, and my sister did all of the camera work. She'd complain, "My shoulder hurts." And I'd shout, "Keep filming!" It was going to be my masterpiece, my homage to Marilyn if you will.

I was heavily invested in the project, which was something of a low-budget Ken Burns knockoff. My sister would zoom in on photos of Marilyn—first with Joe DiMaggio, then with Arthur Miller—and I'd narrate the story. "Her wide eyes, her moist lips, the soft curves of her body," I said, reading off a script I'd typed up, trying to make eye contact with the camera. Later, viewers saw me, an overweight, prepubescent Brad Goreski, drinking ginger ale out of a wineglass—it was supposed to

You're the One That I Want!

GREAT FASHION MOMENTS IN MOVIE MUSICAL HISTORY

Gentlemen Prefer Blondes (1953)

Everyone knows the pink, strapless dress Marilyn wears to sing "Diamonds Are a Girl's Best Friend." But what's maybe even more impressive is the film's opening, where Marilyn and Jane Russell sing "Two Little Girls from Little Rock." The long-sleeved gowns with the plunging neckline make this the most fabulous opening to a movie ever.

Summer Stock (1950)

Judy Garland sings "Get Happy" wearing the iconic blazer with the hat, the hose, and the pumps—every designer has done their version of that look ever since. But it's really about the red lip. And who doesn't love this song? I didn't think you could improve on this song until she and Barbra Streisand did a duet of it on *The Judy Garland Show* in 1963. Perfection.

Cabaret (1972)

Yes, there was Liza Minnelli's amazing performance as Sally Bowles, and the makeup and the hair. But to me, this is all about the green nails. It's such a strange character choice and something that comes up in fashion over and over again. As I write this, it's all about the jade nail. Liza did it first.

West Side Story (1961)

Whenever I try something on and feel beautiful, I want to dance around the dressing room like Natalie Wood as Maria, singing "I Feel Pretty" in that simple white dress.

Grease (1978)

I often feel like Olivia Newton-John's character Sandy, who is reminiscent of Sandra Dee. She's the goody-two-shoes, and so

(CONTINUED ON NEXT PAGE)

put-together with her cardigans. But we all have another side to our personalities—a more daring, sexy side. I've always been obsessed with her at the end of *Grease*. As a kid, I'd wait for that moment when she comes out dressed in the leather jacket and the high-waisted pants with her hair blown out big. Everybody has a wild side, and this is a reference I come back to again and again.

Top Hat (1935)
Ginger Rogers wearing the feather dress, with the perfect flow that floats on air and barely exists in our world? The combination of this light chiffon gown and Ginger Rogers and Fred Astaire dancing together is a match made in heaven. I could watch that dress move as much as I could watch her dance.

be champagne—toasting the actress's glamorous life. The video was all kinds of inappropriate. I styled my cousin as Marilyn, in a wig we had left over from some Halloween costume and an evening dress hanging in my mom's closet, which I don't think she ever wore but was perfect here. I also included a naked photograph of Marilyn. I talked about her rough years in explicit, ridiculous detail. "She did not receive the love that every child receives," I said, "so as a teenager she was a prostitute." A *prostitute*. I felt like a major success that day. Until another girl in class had the audacity to make a video presentation, too. I sat in class thinking, Mine's definitely better.

But Ruby loved the video presentation, not for its aesthetics but for what it represented. Because all Grandma Ruby ever wanted was for me to be myself. She was perceptive in that way—a truth sayer and see-er for both of us Goreski kids. My sister dated a boy in high school, and when they broke up, Ruby said to her, "He wasn't right for you. He never looked me in the eye. He would have held you back."

Everything I Know About Fashion I Learned When I Was Five

PLAYING DRESS-UP ISN'T JUST FOR KIDS

The first question we ask ourselves in the morning is always the same: "What am I going to wear today?" Why is that? Because what we wear is our armor—it announces our identity while protecting us from the stresses life throws at us daily.

I am known for wearing bow ties, and I have something like 150 in my collection. Believe it or not, the bow tie started as a joke. My boyfriend bought me the first one while he was on vacation in London. We were going out one night with some old friends to a straight bar, and I thought I'd test it out, pairing a bow tie with a cardigan and a dress shirt—just to see what the reaction would be. Well, I found it was a conversation piece. In a good way. Strangers were coming up to me all night telling me how much they liked it.

I was living in Los Angeles at the time, and the bow tie became a reaction to the laid-back, casual cool of L.A. It was a way to get noticed in a sea of people all trying to be noticed.

> **Believe it or not, the bow tie started as a joke.**

And something was in the air. Labels like Thom Browne and Band of Outsiders were playing with shrunken proportions, and the bow tie seemed to go along with the playful silhouettes. There was a sense of humor to dressing up that I appreciated. For a while I was wearing tennis sweaters to the office. I'd sit there in a polka-dot tie and tennis whites wondering, Why am I dressed like this? In a way, it was a return to my roots, to the classic American, Ralph Lauren look I wore in the third grade. I realized I was playing a character.

> **It was a way to get noticed in a sea of people all trying to be noticed.**

(CONTINUED ON NEXT PAGE)

That changed the way I approached styling and style: Dressing up isn't just for kids. We're all playing characters—in the office, out with our loved ones. And style inspiration can come from anywhere. The other day I saw a box of Crayola crayons at the supermarket, which later inspired an outfit. I put on a candy-striped, rainbow polo shirt; a navy blazer; white jeans; and bright green high-top sneakers. Some days I wake up and feel like a chorus boy from the movie *Grease*. Some days I'm Danny Zuko, some days I'm Sandra Olsen. After a particularly long week I'm sometimes feeling the sad clown look—pairing a shawl-collared jacket with a sloppy Lanvin bow tie. Life is more fun when you're playing different characters and not locking yourself into a look. Why be the goth girl all the time? Step outside of your comfort zone and don't get locked into a uniform.

> **" Step outside of your comfort zone and don't get locked into a uniform."**

"When I grow up," I told Ruby, "I want to be either a makeup artist or a window dresser." She didn't flinch. Ruby only said, "Be a makeup artist. They make more money."

had less-practical advice from my father. Though he was always around, he spent a lot of time in the garage. He was the kind of dad that was always building something, busy with the table saw. He enjoyed chopping wood in the forest near our house and then falling asleep in a chair in front of the TV. He wasn't some weird mountain man. He was incredibly talented. He built the house we lived in from the ground up. I think part of that was just his wanting to get away from the stresses of home but also wanting to provide a beautiful place for his family to live. It was his way of showing us that he loved us. When he and my mother briefly split up, she went to Toronto and we remained with our father in Apple Valley. When I was getting dressed to go to a family event or a movie, he'd yell up to me from the stuck-in-the-seventies kitchen with its mustard-yellow appliances, "It's not a fashion show! Hurry up!" But he was wrong. For me, every day was a fashion show.

> "For me, every day was a fashion show."

My father didn't care much about what he wore. He had a mustache. He dressed in sweatpants and duck boots and if he was going out at night with my mom, it was polo shirts and blue jeans. There wasn't a lot

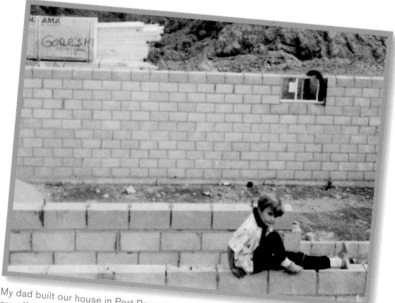

My dad built our house in Port Perry, on a tract of land he bought from my grandfather. This photo is memorable because of the pose: This is the beginning of my trying to find myself as a high-fashion model.

of variation. He was conservative in his beliefs, and quiet, too. With me, anyway. He and my sister seemed to understand each other. He played in a slow-pitch baseball league on Monday nights and my sister went to every game with him up until she went off to university. My mother and I—we had our own routine. On Thursday nights, we'd go food shopping and she'd buy fashion magazines for me, which I smuggled back to my room. Why the secrecy? Yes, my father had taken me trick-or-treating as Madonna. But I think he preferred the illusion. When I was too out front, too obvious with my first loves, he acted out. I came home from school one day to find that my Barbie dolls were gone, and it was no mystery what happened to them. More than once when Grandma Ruby would take me to the toy store, I'd pull a Barbie doll down from the shelf, and she'd smile at me and say, "We'll have to sneak this one."

> "I taught myself to shave. (And to put on a full face, for that matter.)"

My father loved me. I know that. But he didn't always understand me. And frankly, I don't blame him. It was a two-way street. I wasn't emotionally available to him, and I rarely engaged with him. We didn't have anything in common. We never had that sitcom moment, like on *The Cosby Show,* where Dr. Huxtable shows Theo how to shave. I taught myself to shave. (And to put on a full face, for that matter.) He was interested in snowblowers and anything with an on/off switch. Everything he was, I was not. I never felt a lack of love from him. It's just that my mother understood me enough for the both of them. I had such strong female role models in my childhood that I never sought that love and acceptance from him.

I was happiest—or maybe safest—in the basement with my mom. The room had wainscoting running along the bottom of the walls and a border done in muted colors. And we'd sit at her Singer sewing machine in the corner adding plaid patches onto ripped knees. I liked to personalize my clothing even then. The basement was a place where the glue gun was always hot and at the ready. There, I never needed an excuse to put sequins on anything. I later joined the local community theater, and my mom and I would plant ourselves in the basement sewing more and more sequins onto the costumes, sometimes right up until closing night.

My mother encouraged my creativity. There was a period where I wore gymnastic shoes everywhere. I'd taken a jazz dance class, and while the steps didn't stick, the shoes did. I'd put on my Esprit yellow wool V-neck sweater with the gray, mauve, and white argyle print with my Hollywood brand jeans cuffed high. I'd come downstairs and I could see the worry on her face: What was going to happen today? She wasn't interested in stifling my creativity. Far from it. When she asked what kind of curtains I wanted for my bedroom, and I asked for sequined Roman shades, she didn't put up a fight. She didn't suggest something blue and masculine or something with a sports theme. She went to the fabric store and custom-made the sequined window treatments to my specifications. But like all mothers, she wanted her son to be safe. And at school, I wasn't always safe.

My parents had questions—about me, about why I liked Barbie dolls and blondes and Debbie Gibson and why I wasn't growing out of that. They didn't understand why I was dancing and lip-synching to Madonna singles in the living room. For answers, they turned to a doctor.

When I turned twelve and hadn't stopped playing with dolls, my parents took me to see a therapist in Toronto, Dr. Kenneth Zucker, a man who felt if he could diagnose me as a gay, he might be able to cure me. His specialty was gender identity, and he wanted to see if I was confused about what I was. (I wasn't.)

It came on suddenly. One afternoon in the fifth grade, my parents pulled me out of school and drove me into Toronto for what they called "family therapy." We were all going to this doctor, they said, to deal with the recent death of my maternal grandfather, Harry. He and Ruby had gone on a vacation to Portugal and the night they returned, Harry suffered a heart attack. Three days later he passed away.

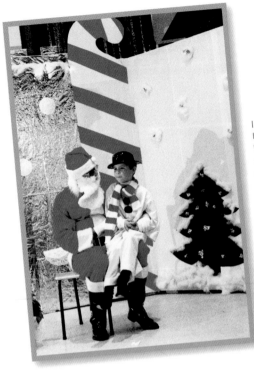

I took jazz lessons at the United Church, and here I am at the Christmas concert. I liked the classes. But I liked the jazz slippers even more, and I wore them around the house forever.

It was a devastating loss for the family and it destroyed my mother and sister. The only other person I knew who had died was my aunt Judy. We probably needed the counseling. The office would provide a safe space to talk—about my grandfather, but also about me and my weight issues. (I was eating my feelings.) We talked about the boys at school and the bullying. And sometimes when Dr. Zucker sat with my parents, I went and saw a medical student, Myra. What she and I did felt more like hanging out than anything more serious. We just talked about what my life was like. She was beautiful, which made it easier to talk. It always comes down to someone being pretty.

But these sessions weren't always so benign. Sometimes it was *me* on display, me seated in front of that two-way mirror, me under observation. Dr. Zucker placed me in one examination room where there was a bucket full of G.I. Joes on one side and a selection of Barbie dolls on the other. He told me he'd be right back, and in the meantime I should go ahead and play with any toys I wished. While my heart desperately wanted to reach for Barbie's shiny blond hair and Ken's waxed chest, I refused to give this doctor the satisfaction. And so I sat with G.I. Joe and pretended I enjoyed plastic warfare; it was the longest hour of my life. It didn't help that the doctor's office on Spadina Avenue looked exactly like you'd expect a 1980s mental health building in downtown Toronto to look. The floors were white, the walls were cream, and the whole thing felt sterile. I like to think my parents knew, on some level, that nothing would change me. We were there because they felt helpless and because my pediatrician recommended we see Dr. Zucker. My parents wouldn't have thought of such a thing on their own. Still, there I was. At night, safely back home, I'd sit on my sister's bed, trying to understand what was happening. "Dr. Zucker asks me weird questions," I said, breaking down in tears.

> "While my heart desperately wanted to reach for Barbie's shiny blond hair and Ken's waxed chest, I refused to give this doctor the satisfaction."

The doctor recommended I spend more time with my father. And so I went to baseball games with him. I chopped wood. I picked rocks out of the new plot of land he bought, so he could build on it. But, like the song goes in *La Cage aux Folles,* I am who I am. People often blame kids who are bullied for bringing this hurt on themselves. *Why can't you just blend in?* they say. *Why attract so much attention to yourself by dressing weird or talking weird?* Well, I tried that. I wasn't wearing faux fur in the fifth grade when that blond He-Man called me names. I was dressed like all the other boys, in starched shirts and collars. But somehow these kids could sniff something different on me, something they didn't like, something they didn't understand. And I could never please them even if I tried. In the third grade, I lip-synched to "Like a Virgin" on Talent

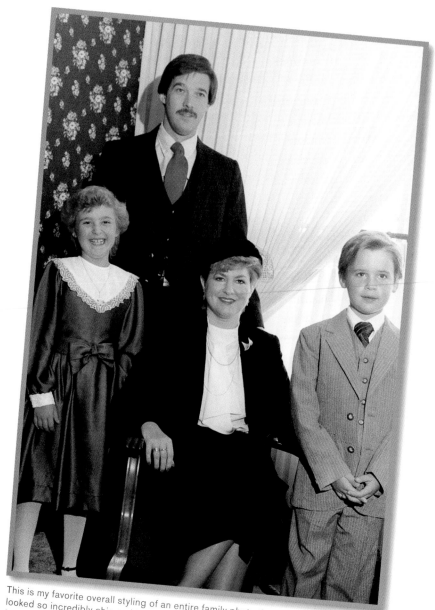

This is my favorite overall styling of an entire family photo that we have. My mom looked so incredibly chic and beautiful on this day. It's one of my favorite outfits of hers. That veil, come on!

Day in class, and I put my Lite-Brite on the floor pointing up at me like a spotlight. I wasn't trying to be brazen. I wasn't trying to stick a big middle finger up to the school. That wasn't the kind of kid I was. I wasn't angry. I was just trying to be myself. I was just the kid who loved Marilyn Monroe, whose definition of beauty was defined by Marilyn, and who liked dancing to Madonna because she was the new Marilyn.

In my fifth-grade class, we had a lip-synching contest every Friday. I have no idea why. Maybe because it was the eighties. The other boys would perform things like Billy Idol's "Mony Mony" and Aerosmith. But I lip-synched to Debbie Gibson's "Out of the Blue." I put a bow in my hair and I borrowed a bubble skirt from a friend and I had little lace socks and running shoes. I was visual, so I enlisted five girls from my class to sit up front and blow bubbles at me while I performed. I wasn't worried what the other boys in class would think of me. I was more concerned that the girls were going to mess up the bubbles. All I could think about was that these girls were going to ruin my act!

That was my childhood. None of it was a response to what the other kids were doing. None of it was a reaction to bullies. I just didn't know any better. No, I didn't know any *different*. I was naïve and aloof and I didn't know how else to be. All I wanted was to turn the lights off in our portable classroom and convince the kids from my class to perform five numbers from the musical *Cats;* for a set we built a pyramid out of milk crates and draped it in old blankets. I had a vision, and even though the trash pile was unstable, and kids were falling off and scraping their knees, we made it work. We wore costumes borrowed from the local community theater. And it was awesome.

> "But somehow these kids could sniff something different on me, something they didn't like, something they didn't understand. And I could never please them even if I tried."

I'm sure my mom knew this whole thing with Dr. Zucker might be detrimental, that it might leave the kind of mark you can't see on the surface but nevertheless festers beneath. At least she knew enough to take me to McDonald's after. McDonald's is where all parents take kids when they feel guilty about something.

Years later, as a college student in Toronto, I would show that video of my Marilyn Monroe presentation to a friend. She and I hadn't talked much about my childhood, and I thought she would laugh. But instead she cried. She saw this cute, chubby, awkward boy showing off his Marilyn Monroe calendar and her heart broke. I didn't need to say a word. She knew the struggles that a boy like this must have endured in high school. She knew this overly sensitive boy's teenage years must have been hell. She had no idea.

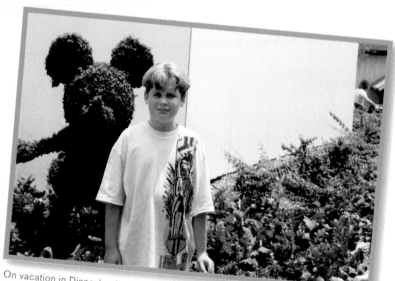

On vacation in Disneyland, my parents bought me an Ocean Pacific T-shirt. To me, this was a major designer label and a true status symbol. It was also the closest I came to dressing masculine and sporty. My hair here loosely resembles Marilyn Monroe's (intentional) and Queen Elizabeth's (unintentional).

2

Anger can be your best friend. Especially when you have no friends.

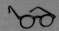

THE FASHION INDUSTRY IS full of people who were not "cool" in high school. People who were misunderstood. People who dressed outlandishly because there was no other way to express themselves. No one had it easy. Lady Gaga—then Stefani Germanotta—was bullied for dressing too provocatively. Even Kate Middleton was called gangly by the girls at her grade school. We were all of us misunderstood. Who knew I'd have something in common with the Princess of Pop and a duchess?

For me, high school was a study in isolation. I was fifteen years old, sitting on my windowsill, beneath the same gold sequined Roman shades my mother made for me. My bedroom was my refuge. I was lighting incense and candles and staring up at the stars, smoking a cigarette out the window, dreaming of a better place. It was high drama! But I lived in fear of going to school. I was superstitious bordering on obsessive-compulsive. I said a prayer in the morning and another at night, asking Him (whoever He is) to watch over me. If I fell asleep before saying the prayer, I was convinced the next day would be tragic.

And let's face it: Sometimes it was. High school is tough, the hallways often cold. A teenager's locker is one of their few chances for self-expression, and I wanted to personalize mine with photos of Calvin

"For me, high school was a study in isolation."

Klein models. But I didn't want to draw any more attention to myself. So I hung photos of the Beastie Boys instead—still personal, because I loved their wit, but less conspicuous. Sometimes I ate lunch in the stairwell with two girlfriends, usually salad I brought with me from home. Or I ate in the school library, even though we weren't supposed to. The teachers didn't have the heart to tell me to go to the cafeteria, because they knew I could no longer walk into the cafeteria without the boys in my class throwing food at me. I can't remember a single day where someone didn't imitate my voice in class. Or call me the F-word in the hallways. The word did hurt, but not because it was a surprise to me. Duh! I knew I was gay the first time I saw the opening credits to *Who's the Boss* and a shirtless Tony Danza opened the shower curtain. The word hurt because it made it all real. It meant I would have to act on those feelings one day soon. And I was scared by what that meant for my life. I didn't have any role models; I didn't have a picture of what a happy, well-adjusted gay couple would look like. I thought being gay meant angry families and loneliness. I was worried about the loneliness. High school—for me and every other teenager since the dawn of time— was a minefield of angst like *My So-Called Life,* except in real life Jared Leto never falls in love with the girl with the Kool-Aid dye job.

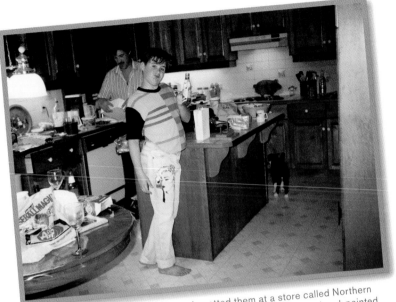

This photograph is all about the jeans. I spotted them at a store called Northern Reflections. And they were expensive—because some crazy queen hand-painted Madonna's face on the right thigh. I begged my mom to buy these for me, which she did. And I wore them everywhere.

I made an effort. I should say this. For exactly two weeks I tried to fit in. I tried to pare it down, to limit the color in every sense. But it didn't feel right. It didn't feel like *me*. Besides, people knew who I was. People knew what I was. I was the kid who plucked his eyebrows so much that there was basically one hair left. One tiny little hair. I was only fooling myself. I cried a lot—

> "I didn't have any role models; I didn't have a picture of what a happy, well-adjusted gay couple would look like."

often because my sister was gone, off to university. She and I had talked about my sexuality before she left. I told her I thought I was gay. Of course I knew I was gay, but I was trying to test the waters, to see what her reaction might be. Any time I got up the courage to float the idea, her answer was always the same: "You'll be what you're gonna be. And you're my brother. It doesn't matter."

If I had an escape in these years—beyond my bedroom windowsill and the basement with the sewing machine and my pictures of Claudia Schiffer and Naomi Campbell—if there was a place where I could be myself, unapologetically, it was theater camp. The summer after tenth grade, I enrolled in a one-week intensive drama program called Theater Ontario. I know that seven days doesn't sound like much time, but the experience was transformative. It wasn't just the classes, though the instruction was impressive, too. I took stage combat lessons and musical theater workshops and worked on monologues and learned to tap dance. But what made more of an impression was the taste of freedom. We kids lived in college dorms and stayed up all night dancing. Not sleeping was a point of pride. We chanted like Buddhists in the courtyard for hours. There was a real hippie vibe to the place and we embraced the free-love spirit. It was a chance for self-expression. There was the gamine girl with the red pixie haircut who wore baby-doll dresses with denim shorts underneath—a heightened nineties look. There was the girl who wore a tailcoat every single day. And the girl who sat in the courtyard with a broken keyboard, playing original songs with gibberish lyrics, and we'd all listen and do interpretive dance. It was all about feeling the moment. That summer I kissed a boy for the first time. His name was Ian, and I knew enough to know I liked it, that it felt right to me. Girls were my friends, not my love interests.

This collection of outsiders at Theater Ontario? The ones who came from local communities that weren't always accepting of them? We were thrilled to have found one another. And so we kept the camp spirit alive during the winter by getting together as often as possible. My friend Victoria—with the big eyes and the chestnut, shoulder-length hair—would come visit me in Port Perry; we'd walk the town's Main Street and she'd laugh. "Why does every store sell potpourri!" she'd say. I couldn't argue with her; she was right. There wasn't much to do in Port Perry, I said. This was the kind of place where teenagers take their pickup trucks out to the cornfield and drink cans of beer in front of a bonfire. It's like *Footloose,* minus the hot Southern boys and the angsty solo dance scene. And so Victoria and I would sit in the Goreski family hot tub in our backyard, pretending we were mermaids. We were bored. We painted our nails black. We ate too much. We called ourselves Fat Brad and Fat Victoria, and we got excited about putting potato chips in our sandwiches.

> "It's like *Footloose,* minus the hot Southern boys and the angsty solo dance scene."

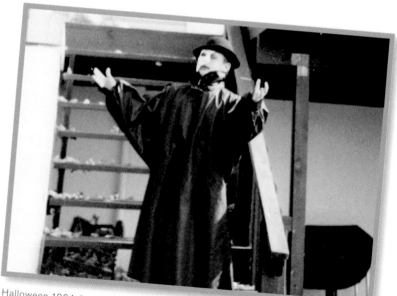

Halloween 1994. I was obsessed with *The Phantom of the Opera.* When it was announced that the musical was coming to Toronto, my grandfather got on the phone immediately and bought tickets for the family.

Reduce, Reuse, Recycle

HOW TO BUY VINTAGE (AND WHEN TO WALK AWAY!)

1. Don't be afraid to get dirty. Sometimes you have to dig deep to find that one precious item. Roll up your sleeves, grab some Purell, and get in there.
2. Know what you are shopping for. Vintage shops and flea markets can be overwhelming. But if you have a direction, you're more likely to find what you're looking for—and maybe, if you're lucky, you'll find some hidden treasures along the way.
3. Point and click. I buy a lot of vintage online at eBay and 1stdibs to give as gifts—especially jewelry. There are some great resources and great deals and you don't have to leave the comfort of your own home. It's always nice to avoid that extra price markup you often find in stores.
4. Do your homework. When you travel, look for local flea markets and ask about the great vintage stores. Each country/city has its own unique pieces, and your purchases will be mementos of your adventures.
5. If the price is right but the item is too big, it's often worth it to make the purchase and then have it altered. Don't leave behind a good find just because it is too big. You may regret it later . . .
6. Let yourself *splurge* on that designer item you're lusting over. I almost left a Chanel briefcase behind in a vintage store in Paris and found myself running back hours later, minutes before closing time. It's one of my fave items I own!

I tried to dye Victoria's hair blond, which high school kids everywhere need to stop doing, by the way. It was a disaster. She'd previously put henna in her hair to give it a reddish tint, and when I applied the bleach the chemicals burned her scalp and ruined the color.

It was more fun when I went into Toronto on the weekends, taking the train to Victoria's apartment, where our camp friends would all descend. Victoria was raised by a single mom, a progressive hippie who didn't much care what we did, and she never asked questions. Friends would come in for auditions and crash at Victoria's two-bedroom. You never had to give much notice. You'd call on a Friday night and say, "I'm getting on the train. I'll be at Union Station at ten. OK?" And it was. It was a lot of slumber parties and all-ages rock shows and tickets to Lollapalooza. We'd go to the theater. We'd go shopping on Queen Street, stopping into Black Market for vintage T-shirts and going to the Goodwill store, where you could buy clothes and pay by the pound. Looking back on it, buying used clothing in bulk sounds pretty gross. But for a teenager with no money, there was nothing better than walking out of a store with a couple pounds of new clothing. It made us feel rich. It was a beautiful time capsule. Best of all, at Victoria's apartment, it wasn't just that I could be gay. I could *talk* about it. Out loud. Victoria was "of the city." She was one of the first people I met where I thought, I don't need to have any secrets with you.

This was the nineties. Kurt Cobain had passed away and I'd gotten into the grunge scene. I was often angry in these years. Unable to channel my frustrations into words, I expressed myself through fashion, just like I had as an eleven-year-old pretending to be Don Johnson at my communion. I started listening to the Breeders and Nine Inch Nails and Smashing Pumpkins and I stopped wearing penny loafers. I fell under the spell of the Seattle movement, and I wasn't alone. In 1992 I remember watching Marc Jacobs on *Fashion Television* talking about the grunge collection he designed for Perry Ellis—the daring line that got him fired from the venerable label. Steven Meisel photographed that flannel collection for *Vogue* in a legendary shoot with Naomi Campbell, Nadja Auermann, and Kristen McMenamy. I tore those pages out of the magazine, savoring the images of Kristen with that pageboy haircut and the beat-up purple Doc Martens and the leather jacket and flannel shirt tied around her waist. It was the antithesis of everything I'd worn before and I loved it. I kept these magazine clippings in a file (which my dad still has). I kept all of the Guess ads, because I was obsessed with Claudia Schiffer—another sort of neo–Marilyn Monroe. I grew my hair long, dyed it auburn and then jet-black.

> "I was often angry in these years. Unable to channel my frustrations into words, I expressed myself through fashion."

Grunge fashion was my armor. I was Ally Sheedy on the outside but Molly Ringwald on the inside. We were listening to Hole and angry Seattle noise. And we were experimenting with alcohol, and later with marijuana. We were leaving Victoria's apartment after midnight and not coming home until the sun came up. We were part-time club kids, too, plain and simple, and to me it was all very glamorous. We'd board a bus that would take us to a secret location. It was always some secret location and we'd end up God knows where in a warehouse and dancing all night with pacifiers and whistles and candy necklaces around our necks.

For me, rave culture was all about the clothing. It was a chance to dress up and play a character—in the same way I did at Halloween. At vintage stores, I drew my inspiration not just from *Vogue* but also from a *Geraldo* episode on New York club kids. I wore knee-high socks and terry-cloth shorts and skintight T-shirts and a see-through

> "Grunge fashion was my armor. I was Ally Sheedy on the outside but Molly Ringwald on the inside."

Pocahontas knapsack. At Victoria's apartment, I could play dress-up all the time. I could listen to gay house music we bought on cassette and put on a sailor costume and sequins and let Victoria paint fake tattoos on my arms. When I'd been into grunge, my hair was long and always a different color. Now I chopped it all off. Victoria and I would buy Bingo Dabber—it was almost like puffy paint, the kind bingo players used to ink up their cards.

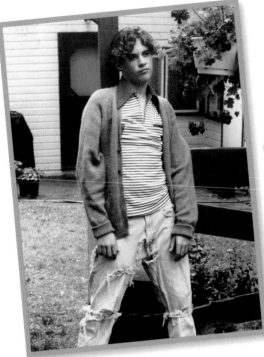

Me in my grunge days.

But we put it in our hair. We'd squeeze the tube against our heads, and it would look like we had full pink plastic helmets on. It was major. I'd come home on Sundays covered in glitter and sleep straight through until Monday morning.

Oh, and it was all on television. Long before *The Rachel Zoe Project,* I was on *Electric Circus,* Canada's Friday-night dance show, which aired on Citytv. I was a minor celebrity in my town because of it. My dad would make fun of the show, calling it "Electric Titties," because there were always close-up shots of women's breasts bouncing on camera. But we loved it. I wore a leopard-print pullover that I found at a vintage store and Victoria and I went to the TV studio, where we sometimes danced with a cartoonlike character dressed in a Winnie-the-Pooh backpack who went

> "I'm sorry," I said, still dancing. "I love this shirt. It sparkles!"

by the name Hot Girl. He looked like Tweedledee from *Alice in Wonderland,* missing Tweedledum. Victoria wore her hair in two buns at the top of her head like Björk. We danced for hours, in these studied movements—we'd punch the air and flail our arms. We didn't care about anything. There, we felt alive.

It was an absurd scene. *Electric Circus* was filmed in the same studio where the eleven o'clock news and the early morning shows were broadcast. We'd be dancing on the same platforms the morning news anchor would use to demonstrate the latest health food cooking trends. We were often on the second floor, only visible in wide shots, and the music was hard to hear. We just felt a bumping bass in the floor. Victoria would say to me, "Are they playing La Bouche?" I'd say, "I think it's 'Everything but the Girl.'" Sometimes the cameras did come upstairs, and the show's host, Monika Deol, would interview some of the dancers live on air. One night, she was talking to my friend Matt up on a platform. He had blue hair. "Is this your first time here?" she asked him. Matt was mumbling, but he managed to get a few words out, telling the host that Victoria and I had brought him to *Electric Circus* and it was his first time. Monika pointed down at me dancing in the crowd. I was dressed in a sequined green oversize blouse and green velvet bell-bottoms. And I had a choker around my neck, made of sequined material left over from community theater shows.

> "This was just another instance in my life where I could see where the party was, but I couldn't figure out how to get there."

"I want your shirt!" she yelled down to me—on Canadian television.

"I'm sorry," I said, still dancing. "I love this shirt. It sparkles!"

Though Victoria and I were often in the crowd at *Electric Circus,* we were never the cool kids—even there. We used to hand out flyers for clubs.

Her Madgesty

WHAT YOU CAN LEARN FROM MADONNA

Some people forget—I don't—but Madonna was the first female pop star to challenge people's thinking on sex and sexuality. She pushed her audience to be brave and bold not just in their fashion choices but also in their lifestyle choices. And to be more accepting, which was so important for me growing up. It was a different era for celebrities, because they were so much less accessible. You had to wait for the TV interview or the magazine to come out to see what Madonna was up to. There was no stylist yet. You didn't know what Madonna was going to do at the MTV Video Music Awards in advance. You had to tune in for the surprise and the drama. The night she performed "Vogue" with the Marie Antoinette costumes and powdered wigs—it was brilliant but so scandalous at the time. Her dancers were gay and overtly sexual. And there was this undercurrent of danger. She was pushing the boundaries, never more so than in the "Justify My Love" video, which I bought on VHS. I had to hide it from my parents, but it was worth it. Here were men kissing and transvestites and breasts. She was everything.

We weren't paid to do this, we didn't get a kickback on the admissions, but handing out those flyers made us feel like a part of something, which is all we wanted. It made us feel like we belonged. More than once, the producers of *Electric Circus* asked Victoria and me to dance in the window—behind a sheet. We'd be the dancing silhouettes, featured players except that you wouldn't be able to see our faces, which was the whole point of being on television. We wanted to be seen! And we were furious. "We're not coming back if we're in the windows," I shouted. This was just another instance in my life where I could see where the party was, but I couldn't figure out how to get there. Of course, we came back the next week. And the week after that. We had to! Because we wanted to be invited to the big, annual *Electric Circus* dance party in Ottawa in the dead of winter. The producers always chose the coolest dancers to go. Try as we did, we were never invited.

I'd started bringing some of Toronto back to Port Perry with me. One night, after a long weekend dancing in Toronto, I invited Lina Love to dinner. Lina Love (not her real name) was a go-go dancer I met at the clubs. The go-go dancers were like celebrities and my dream was to be one of them. They were glamorous in their own way, and Lina was no exception. She had fluorescent yellow hair and no eyebrows. She wore platform shoes and bell-bottoms and booty shorts and crazy knee-high socks and basically looked like an alien. She danced like an anime character, with these weird, robotic movements. I was obsessed with her. She was a real woman, but she looked like a drag queen.

How was dinner that night in Port Perry? Let me just tell you this: My grandparents met Lina Love. On the train back from Toronto, I was freaking out about what they'd say when I brought this Japanese robot to supper. But, I swear to God, my grandfather was so happy I brought a girl home—any girl!—that he welcomed Lina Love to come back anytime. I was so weirded out by the whole thing that I grabbed her hand and took her down to the basement to play dress-up. I wanted her to see these ladybug costumes my mom made for the community theater, which I thought would make excellent rave costumes.

If I was dressing more outlandishly now, it's because I was trying to work out who I was. I was the same Brad Goreski who danced to Debbie Gibson. Only I'd gotten more creative. I dyed my hair purple. I wore Fun Fur pants to school in grade eleven. I used my mom's sewing machine to make my own pants in weird fabrics. One pair was a cotton print of vacuum cleaners. (That is a fashion don't, by the way.) The pants were basically two flour sacks with a drawstring waist, and I'd wear them with a

T-shirt I bought at the Spin Doctors concert all under a peacoat with a fur collar from the Goodwill. I'd stand in garbage pails and have people take my photo. I was a difficult teenager, acting out in other ways. If I wanted the car, I took the car. My mom would tell me not to, and then she'd hear the sound of the garage door opening. She confronted me once—about the late nights out, about the partying. I was so angsty I shouted back, "I don't fucking care what you think." Of that time in my life, she would say I was out of reach. Years later I found out that she would sleep with the portable phone in her hand, which crushed me. But I didn't blame her.

My parents had stopped indulging me with clothing and told me I needed to get a job. For a brief time, I returned to the restaurant at my grandparents' resort, selling ice cream to tourists for four Canadian dollars. But when a job opened up at the local video store I jumped at the chance. The video store was a lifeline to the outside world. And it's where I discovered the documentary *Unzipped.* Doug Keeve is the filmmaker, and he spent a year following Isaac

> "I always thought of the fashion world as a fantasy, make-believe place. But thanks to *Unzipped,* I could see it, I could hear the paper dolls talk."

Mizrahi as the designer was preparing his spring 1994 collection. The movie goes way beyond fly-on-the-wall footage. You're in a fitting with a young, brassy Naomi Campbell, who is complaining about having to take her belly button piercing out. She is gorgeous—just like the photo I had of her hanging on my wall, the one from *Harper's Bazaar,* where Naomi has straight black hair and is dressed in a Jean Paul Gaultier saddle-harness skirt and bustier. Except here she's talking! She's real! Cindy Crawford, Linda Evangelista, Kate Moss, a brand-new Amber Valletta—they're all there in this movie. It's so chic. For his runway show, Mizrahi has this idea to put up a scrim, like at the ballet, so that the audience will be able to see the backstage area during the runway show, even while the models are

Net-à-Porter

LOAD UP YOUR NETFLIX QUEUE WITH THE TEN BEST MOVIES FOR FASHION INSPIRATION

Mahogany (1975)

This is high seventies glamour at its best. Forget the story for a second, which is absurd: Diana Ross is a secretary who is discovered by a modeling agent and becomes a huge high-fashion model before she gets into a car accident. What *Mahogany* is really about: hair sculptures (!) and vintage posing. There is energy in Diana Ross's fingertips.

Sixteen Candles (1984)

Jake Ryan has been a fashion inspiration for my entire life; he made button-down shirts, khakis, and boat shoes sexy. And Molly Ringwald is the epitome of eighties approachable glamour.

Ocean's Eleven (2001)

This is the rare movie where the men's clothing is stronger than the women's. This is a lesson in tailoring and how to look slick without looking cheesy. It's also Brad Pitt at his best.

American Gigolo (1980)

How hot is Richard Gere in this movie? Every. Single. Outfit. This film is about male sexuality—it's about denim shirts and jeans, and being sexy without showing any skin. Which is really what Richard Gere's appeal was anyway. He was never the guy running around shirtless. He had swagger before anybody else did. Rent this film. Or just check out the Herb Ritts photo from this period of Richard Gere with his hands behind his head. Heaven.

Paris Is Burning (1990)

This is a documentary about drag queens living in New York in the late eighties, competing in these downtown late-night balls, each one part of a house. The House of Labasia. The House of Chanel. This was the birth of voguing, which Madonna borrowed and turned into "Vogue." Most of these people didn't have any money. Their lives were a testament to the fact that you can use what you have around you to create something beautiful. We get lost in the idea that everything has to be Gucci, Balenciaga, Prada. But where style inspiration so often comes from is when people have to make it happen for themselves. There was such a sense of community in this film, and a passion for fashion.

La Dolce Vita (1960)
Nothing beats a man in an Italian-made suit. Or a woman dancing in a fountain. End of story.

Clueless (1995)
Pleated plaid miniskirts, oversize belts, platform shoes—this is a lesson in high nineties fashion. Plus, there's a monster makeover in the middle of the movie, which makes it essential viewing.

Truth or Dare (1991)
Where to begin? With the Gaultier costumes? Or with Madonna shopping at Chanel in Paris, where she calls down to the salesclerk and mocks her. She wore a Chanel necklace to give my favorite speech—when she lands in Rome and addresses her fans about the ban the Vatican has put on her show. She keeps screaming, "*Basta!*" at the crowd, but they won't stay quiet.

The Umbrellas of Cherbourg (1964)
A young Catherine Deneuve in France, dressed in flats and shift dresses with bows in her hair—dainty, French, and proper, shot during the time she and Yves Saint Laurent became close. Oh, and it's a musical!

(CONTINUED ON NEXT PAGE)

The Talented Mr. Ripley (1999)

This film had a huge impact on my personal style. But let's focus on Gwyneth Paltrow. Whether she was dressed in a pressed white shirt and full skirt belted or an evening wear look with a black strapless gown and white gloves, a necklace, and earrings with her hair swept up, she was the personification of gorgeous.

HONORABLE MENTIONS

Pretty in Pink (1986)
The Great Gatsby (1974)
Flashdance (1983)
Saturday Night Fever (1977)
Funny Face (1957)
Elizabeth (1998)
A Single Man (2009)
Boogie Nights (1997)
Annie Hall (1977)

changing. At first, the girls are freaking out. They're standing behind the scrim saying, "Can you see me naked?" But you know they love it.

I always thought of the fashion world as a fantasy, make-believe place. But thanks to *Unzipped,* I could see it, I could hear the paper dolls talk. But in a way, it made this world feel even farther away. How does anyone get there? How does anyone fit in?

My father and I weren't talking about *Unzipped.* While he hadn't taught me to shave, he *did* teach me to drive. These were the times that we laughed together. We got into the car one afternoon for a driving lesson and there was a bucket of Kentucky Fried Chicken sitting in the backseat, left over from the night before. As I was backing out of the driveway, my dad reached into the bucket to grab a snack, and my mom and sister were screaming at him from the porch, shouting, "Don't eat that!"

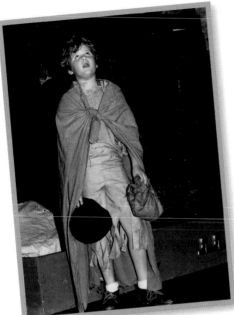

In 1988, I played the title role in *Oliver!* with the Scugog Choral Society and immediately fell in love with acting.

In high school, I landed the lead role in *The King and I*. The director wanted me to shave my head for the role, but I refused. I didn't want to look like Yul Brynner. I wanted to put my own spin on it, which I did, by dyeing my hair black and pulling it into a ponytail. The king was supposed to be hyper-masculine, but I basically dressed like Liza Minnelli.

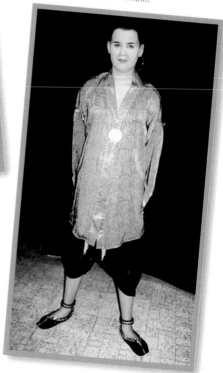

While my dad and I never developed that shorthand that fathers and sons have, he showed his affection in his own way—not through words, but through plywood. In high school, I was heavily involved in the local community theater, and he helped build all of our often-complicated sets. This was nothing like *Waiting for Guffman*. We performed full-length adult shows in the town hall, next to the mayor's house, and our shows ran for two weeks, with several hundred people at each performance. I played all the big roles. I was Billy Bigelow in *Carousel,* dressed in a yellow sweater and a newsboy cap. I was Nicely-Nicely Johnson in *Guys and Dolls.* I played the king of Siam in *The King and I*—with a full face of makeup, including contouring on my nose and eyes to give me an Asian profile.

The theater became an unlikely rallying point for my family. At home, life might have been challenging sometimes. But at the theater we were like the Waltons. My mom made costumes for the theater—exquisite, beautiful costumes that were labors of love. My father worked on pyrotechnics. When I played the Cowardly Lion in *The Wizard of Oz,* sitting for hours in makeup, my mom built the costumes and my father built Oz. When my sister was home from university, she'd double as my personal assistant, running out to get me dinner and bringing me throat lozenges. (Why the lozenges? Because I saw Madonna in *Truth or Dare,* and I wanted the same manic vibe and desperate eleventh-hour emergencies backstage that she thrived on.)

> "I broke down crying. I'm afraid I'm never going to fall in love."

The sound of applause was some much-needed validation of my self-worth. It always had been—since I first stepped onstage at age eleven, in a school play, *The Wild Kingdom,* and then in a local production of *Oliver!* I'll never forget when the director called to say I was cast in the lead role, playing the orphan who dares to ask, "Please, sir, can I have some more?" The whole experience—singing "Where Is Love?," being photographed for the town newspaper—was like me asking for more. It was me asking for more from life.

Working on these shows later provided the kind of quiet moments that I needed with my mom. Even when I was being a brat, we still had to sit together at the sewing machine building the costumes. One night she and I were working on the lion's mane for *The Wizard of Oz* when I got up the nerve to talk to her. To really talk. I was eighteen years old and in my final year of high school. I was waiting for the right moment, but sometimes you have to make the right moment for yourself. For me, that moment was at seven thirty right after *Jeopardy!* ended. I was in the basement with my mom and the fireplace was going. Sewing was a calming influence on her, which I figured would help.

"I think I'm gay," I said to her.

"I know," she said, looking up but not for too long. "Is there anything you're afraid of?"

I broke down crying. "I'm afraid I'm never going to fall in love."

She asked that I not tell my father just yet. That I wait for a time just like this with him where I could connect with him. Unfortunately, that time never came. I never had the opportunity to tell my dad face-to-face that I was gay. Almost a year later, he found out from my cousin, whom I was living with at the time. This was definitely not the way I'd pictured coming out to my dad. I wish he could have heard it from me.

To say I was looking forward to graduation would be a classic understatement. I was tired of running. I wanted out so badly that I almost didn't go to my graduation. And I chose a time-honored night of teenage angst to confront my school demons head-on. I chose the prom.

Believe it or not, my best friend, Tracy Doyle, and I somehow became the outspoken heads of the prom committee. I'd met Tracy on the first day of high school, standing outside of history class. I was wearing a color-blocked Polo rugby—red, blue, green, and yellow—and a white collar. I was still in my preppy phase. Tracy was tall and blond and dressed head-to-toe in an all-black look from Le Château, my favorite gay mall store. She had a wide black headband on her head and was dressed in a gypsy blouse, A-line with bell sleeves that hung over her hands. Everyone else in our class

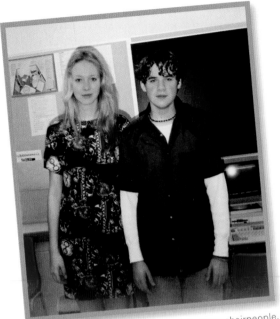

Tracy Doyle and Brad Goreski, unlikely prom chairpeople.

was wearing white T-shirts from the Gap. But there was Tracy, looking like Lady Miss Kier from Deee-Lite.

"You're way too pretty to be in this town," I said. What I meant was that I recognized something in this girl, something I saw in me, too: that our dreams were somehow bigger than this town. We both felt destined to escape. Everyone around us just wanted to make the hockey team and graduate from high school. But we wanted to be heard. We wanted to make our mark beyond the shores of Lake Scugog. We were fast friends, Tracy and I, and everything we did was theatrical, from the school drama club down to the presentations we did in class, which were always as much about the aesthetic as the subject matter. For an English class project, Tracy dressed up as a flapper and did the Charleston.

When it came time for prom committee elections, Tracy and I ran on a ticket of opulence. We figured all of the reasons that people hated us—our bold music taste, our outlandish clothing—were the same reasons we'd put on a good prom. Even our small-minded classmates had to recognize that. We thought it would be fun to plan a party with a real budget and to make something beautiful. We weren't New York trust-fund kids. We were in Ontario on a budget, trying to make something magical happen. And we'd stay up late at Tracy's house, baking pizzas at three in the morning in her kitchen with the marigold curtains that looked like a faded Polaroid, listening to Depeche Mode and Sarah McLachlan's *Fumbling Towards Ecstasy* and dreaming up ways to make the night bigger. The theme was "A Night on the Orient Express," and we imagined this amazing around-the-world tour. We'd dress the gym as Paris! We'd convert the hallways into a Turkish market! Forget the fact that the actual Orient Express didn't travel to most of the places we came up with. This was our prom.

Prom night was my first styling job. Tracy asked me to dress her, and while there weren't yet fashion publicists for me to call, I took it seriously. Tracy and I went to the mall to scout options, browsing the racks at Le Château. After considering many options we bought a knockoff Gianni Versace apron dress like the one Christy Turlington wore in the pages of *Vogue*. I was obsessed with Versace—everything seemed so new, and what he did was the definition of sexy and high fashion. It was so inspirational. And Tracy fit the criteria for a Versace girl—she was tall, thin, and blond, another Barbie in my life. I thought, If I was a girl going to the prom, I'd want to be in Versace and look like Christy Turlington, in a dress inspired by farmer's overalls but with big medallion closures and a pocket on the front. It was a no-brainer. When we got to Tracy's house, she tried the silver metallic dress on for her grandmother, who was horrified by the too-short length and promptly pulled out her sewing machine to add a two-inch lace border. Despite her addition, the dress was perfect. And we found just the right open-toed silver metallic shoes to match. They were a

My Super-Sweet Prom

HOW TO DRESS FOR HIGH SCHOOL'S BIG NIGHT OUT—IN SEVEN SIMPLE STEPS

1. Keep your options open.
I know the dream is to wear a gown. But consider wearing a cocktail-length dress. It's a good way of standing out in the crowd.

2. Be resourceful.
Don't go where everyone else is going. Check out the vintage stores, or even the Goodwill. You never know what you'll find.

3. Pick a decade.
Choose a time period that resonates with you.

4. Be age appropriate.
Girls tend to dress a little risqué for the prom. But you're going to be looking at this photo for the rest of your life. Make sure you don't look "inexpensive." And I'm not talking about how much money you're spending.

5. Do your homework.
What red carpet looks resonate with you? What actress does it well? Who do you want to emulate? Go from that point, instead of wandering around the store being frustrated.

6. Don't be competitive.
That's not what the prom is about. Go shopping with your girlfriends. Make it something fun. Do fittings with each other.

7. Beware of prom hair.
It doesn't have to be overdone. For hair and makeup inspiration, look at magazines. If you're going for a sixties look and you want to do a cat eye and a red lip, I get it. But look at references. Don't be overdone.

size too small, and so on the afternoon of the prom we soaked Tracy's feet in water, shrinking them just enough to squeeze into the shoes. I had to warn her: Listen up, Cinderella, there will be no taking these shoes off at the prom, even for a minute. Because you'll never get them back on.

As for my own wardrobe, I wasn't going to wear a tuxedo to the prom. That much was clear. I had a vision, and it involved a purple Fun Fur jacket. My mom agreed to make this for me, using a men's suit pattern she found in a book and some fake fur she bought at Fabric Land. I'd pair this jacket with a silver lamé ladies' mock turtleneck I found at a used clothing store and a pair of black stretch cigarette pants that looked like they were made from neoprene but were probably acrylic. My shoes were the pièce de résistance: They were DIY two-tone platforms I made in my mom's kitchen by gluing different-colored dime-store flip-flops together and affixing them to the bottom of a pair of patent-leather Converse sneakers. I looked like Michael Alig meets Max Headroom, riding Rainbow Brite. I had to laugh years later when Miuccia Prada did basically the same thing with a line of platform wing tips for men. Some things never go out of style. I bought five pairs of them.

> **"I wasn't going to wear a tuxedo to the prom. . . . I had a vision, and it involved a purple Fun Fur jacket."**

My mom came home and had a fit. Not because I was wearing homemade platform shoes, but because I'd ruined her kitchen to make them. The residue from the glue gun was burned into her brand-new kitchen island—a white ceramic countertop she'd just paid to have installed—and she started to cry. I sensed danger and ran out the back door, my weird platform flip-flops clacking below me.

"You ruined my kitchen!" she shouted after me.

I shouted back, "You ruined my prom! You ruin everything!"

The prom was an epic race to the finish. We worked fourteen-hour days, but surveying the work I felt it was time well spent. My father and I didn't talk much about my two-tone platforms or my silver top, but we did talk about the prom decorations. He agreed to help make some of our elaborate concepts happen. And I appreciated that he recognized this night was important to me and that he volunteered to see it through. The week of the prom, I think he was at the school more than I was. His handiwork was genius. The students would enter the gymnasium through an Egyptian pyramid and there were hieroglyphics on the walls and you could sign your name. There was a spice market where you could get a drink. In another gymnasium down the hall there was a fifteen-foot-tall replica of the Eiffel Tower strung up with Christmas lights (long before Rose Byrne did the same in

> **"I was no longer asking these people to accept me but rather I was announcing myself as someone worth loving."**

Bridesmaids but after Goldie Hawn did it in *Overboard*). We hung two hundred stars from the ceiling, illuminated by black lights. And when the stars didn't glow exactly as planned, we spent $100 on orange and yellow fluorescent spray paint.

But the night wasn't really about the Eiffel Tower. Tracy and I joked about how no one would care what the decorations looked like. That they'd be too drunk to appreciate the craftsmanship. In the end, I was the one who was too drunk. As the head of the prom committee, I had to stand on the front steps of the school greeting my classmates as they entered. I was scared out of my mind. But also proud that I'd made it this far, despite them. I wanted to stare down these people as they entered the prom. I wanted to announce my independence from them, from the long arm of their small-minded bullying. I was no longer asking these people to accept me but rather I was announcing myself as someone worth loving. No one could touch me that night. No one could disrespect me.

Flanked by the school principal and vice principal, trying to hide the fact that I was drunk on lemon gin and Sprite, I stood my ground. Rorschach tests and gender-identity quizzes? I wish Dr. Zucker had just taught me to have a little confidence. I would have been much better off.

It was time to leave. I was headed to university in the fall. I didn't know what I wanted. I didn't know who I was. And that was OK. I saw my name in lights—the lights of a Broadway marquee. And I was going to theater school to play dress-up, to try that life on for size.

In so many ways, this was only the beginning.

3

Never adopt a fashion trend while on vacation. Or how running away can sometimes be the answer to your problems.

HAVE YOU SEEN A *Chorus Line*? Maybe I should start there. You know the character Diana Morales, the Puerto Rican girl? The one so terribly underestimated by all of her teachers? Well, she sings this song called "Nothing," about this improvisation class where her teacher says to the students, "You're a bobsled. It's snowing out. And it's cold. Okay! GO!" They're told to be a table, be a sports car. Be an ice cream cone.

Well, I soon found out, that's *exactly* what theater school is really like. And I loved it. I was nineteen years old and living on my own for the first time, studying at the conservatory of musical theater training at George Brown College. While it wasn't exactly Juilliard, George Brown promised to prepare a generation of actors for a life in the theater. We were in workshops eight hours a day, six days a week, and the instructors were not shy about weeding out those of us who didn't have a future onstage. There were thirty of us in my class and less than half of us would graduate. The program was that intense.

And there I was, feeling exactly like Diana Morales in *A Chorus Line,* when my teacher said, "You are an egg. Pretend you are an egg and you are about to hatch. Go!"

It was not glamorous. The school was housed in a nondescript 1950s building in the Casa Loma neighborhood of Toronto. George Brown was a technical college, and our classes were held in the basement, in the same rooms where aspiring plumbers and refrigerator maintenance students convened. We shared one classroom with the upholstery department, and we were regularly asked to move out half-built, torn-apart furniture to make room for our dance classes. The school has since hooked up with a local theater company, the Soulpepper Theatre, and the George Brown drama students now study in a state-of-the-art facility with beautiful dance studios and black box theaters. But us? We just had upholstery. There were some kids who took it way too seriously. We'd walk into vocal class, and they would have been there for forty-five minutes, getting their bodies warm. These are the people who were rehearsing lines in the hallway, mumbling to themselves. The ones who looked down on us for being silly. But some of it was silly! The boys would be in the bathroom, changing into their dance belts and tights for ballet class. I loved the juxtaposition of these guys jamming their junk into a pair of tights next to the plumber taking a pee. And then there I was, running down the halls doing leaps in my tights.

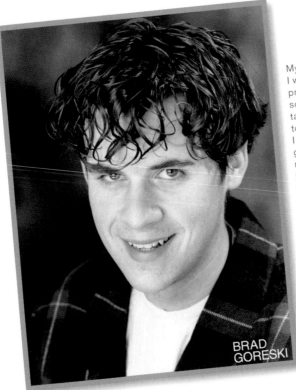

My first headshots! I wanted to be a professional actor, and so I had these photos taken and then sent them to all of the big agencies I could find in Toronto. I got one response from a major agency. It wasn't the response I was hoping for. The woman wrote to say that the agency wasn't taking on any new clients, but she had a few suggestions for me. First, I should put less product in my hair. Second, I should wear more makeup. How dare she!

BRAD GORESKI

And it was fantasy land, an extension of theater camp and those late-night raves and the community theater troupe back in Port Perry. Here, I took voice lessons and Shakespeare classes. I was still playing dress-up, only now the clothes fit. I'd lost twenty-five pounds since high school, thanks in part to cutting meat and pepperoni sticks and deep-fried Oreos out of my diet, and I was feeling good. I was a serious student, and I was determined to be one of the success stories. I was thrilled when the school felt the same way. My first written report card offered a hint of promise. It read, "You are the embryo for a fine actor." Me! An embryo!

Lighten Up

HOW I LOST TWENTY-FIVE POUNDS—AND KEPT IT OFF

As a kid, I was overweight and creative—a terrible combination, because I had a habit of turning snacking into an elaborate art project. For a special treat, I'd sometimes scrape the icing from the inside of a dozen Oreo cookies; roll the white, sugary goodness into a ball of confectionery joy; and freeze it for later. My mom says when I was a baby, one of the first things she noticed about me was that I growled for food. I scared her the first time she heard it. I was eight months old, sitting in a high chair at a restaurant, growling at the staff as they walked by. And so my mom resorted to bringing crackers with her everywhere we went just to keep me quiet—the crackers acted like some carbohydrate pacifier. I love food. Always have and always will. But for me, everything is about balance and moderation. Here are a few things I do to keep my weight down.

1. Eat well!

Eating well starts with a high-protein, low-carb, low-sugar diet. Steel-cut oats, nonfat Greek yogurt, fruit, vegetables, lean proteins, not too much added salt or oils. It doesn't sound fun, but it tastes great and keeps my energy up.

2. Get moving.

Exercise: I know, not a revolutionary concept. But not only does it keep the weight off, but it also helps you clear your mind. I don't work out for hours either. Forty-five minutes to one hour is more than enough time to get the endorphins pumping.

3. Go ahead and cheat.

If I want a cupcake or French fries from time to time, I indulge. At my house, we have pizza every Sunday. It's a tradition! But try to eat cheat foods earlier in the day. It makes a difference.

4. Walk it off.
I travel a lot. If I can't work out at the hotel gym, I'll try to walk instead of taking a cab. Or I'll take the stairs instead of the elevator (within reason). I also go out dancing a lot. I consider that cardio.

Onstage, I was experimenting with form and style. Offstage, I was experimenting with my sense of self, which seems to be what college is all about. I took my studies seriously. I was barely even drinking. Until one night when I was on the way back from a weekend away in Montreal with some school friends. There was a horrific ice storm, and I actually thought we were going to die. The ice was coming down in sheets. When we got into Toronto, I was just happy to be alive. It was a Friday night and to celebrate our return we went out dancing. But I was still so shaken that when a friend offered me a line of cocaine, I thought, What the hell.

It's funny. Back in high school, I'd made the mistake of telling my sister about the first time I smoked pot. She looked at me and shook her head, saying, "Bradley, this is just the beginning." At the time, I laughed. I mean, it was so Afterschool Special of her. But that night I heard those words ringing in my head and I thought, Maybe she was right.

Freshman year passed in a blur and I stayed in Toronto for the summer. I couldn't imagine returning to Port Perry, not when I'd tasted city life. To pay my bills, I got a summer job working in retail. "Hi, welcome to the Gap." The door greeter? Yeah, that was me, in the summer of 1997 in Toronto. I liked my coworkers well enough but I hated the job. I hated the fluorescent lighting. I always made my sales quota but let's face it, this was a summer job. I knew my heart wasn't in it. One day, I called my boss to say I wasn't coming in.

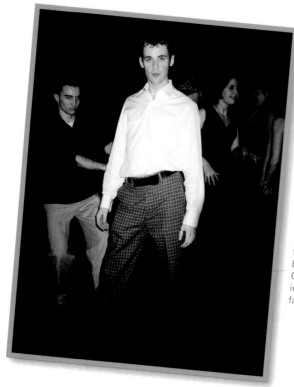

Christmas 1996. I'm wearing Club Monaco pants that are way too big for me. I've got a belt on, yet it doesn't look like it's even cinching anything. And then there are the platform boots and my famous Caesar haircut. All in all, this is a big fashion don't!

"Remember that audition I told you about?"

"No," he said.

"Well, I got it! And it's filming today!"

Of course there was no audition. There was no acting job. But I'd been out all night and I couldn't bring myself to get up from bed. I was folding chinos at the Gap during the day, but at night I was hanging out at the drag clubs in Toronto. And I developed definite opinions about which queens were talented and which ones were phoning it in. I had no time for the queens who didn't bother to learn the lyrics, who stood onstage mouthing *"apples, pears, and peaches"* in time with the music. Frankly, as a theater student I was offended. By the way, everything I know about drag—from tucking, to shading, to contouring the bridge of the nose—I learned from RuPaul's book *Lettin It All Hang Out,* which I read in my first year of college when I had mono.

Life that summer was a big party. But when I returned to school in the fall, the party didn't stop.

I quit working at the Gap and found a job waiting tables at Five Doors North, an Italian restaurant on Yonge Street. The restaurant was so cool there wasn't even a sign outside. You had to know about it to find it, which I loved. The food there was delicious—inexpensive, small plates for people to share—and I think the owners kept it reasonably priced so people would drink more wine, which they did. It was a party atmosphere at the restaurant, for the customers and the staff, too. It was around this time that Whitney Houston was in the first throes of her abuse, and we had a wall in the kitchen where we hung up newspaper clippings of her awesome exploits. People would come in to see the "Whitney Wall of Shame." I was working with a bunch of lost souls. But they were lost souls I loved being around. Every night felt like a performance. And sometimes it was. I'd get up on the bar and lip-synch to Jennifer Holliday, usually while the restaurant was still packed with customers. One night I grabbed

Sashay! *Chantez!*

WHAT YOU CAN LEARN FROM DRAG QUEENS

Drag queens live in a universe of heightened glamour—the hair is big, the lashes are long, and the sequins are extra sparkly. They offer us an insight into their ideas of femininity, sexuality, and humor. It's about creating a character, dressing up, living your fantasy in front of others. Drag queens own who they are, and more important, they are fashion trailblazers and fantastic creative minds. A constant source of inspiration!

a super-straight guy's motorcycle helmet and did runway down the bar. I told everyone I was in the Alexander McQueen show.

And for the first time in my life, I was making good money. I used to walk around this great department store, Holt Renfrew—Toronto's answer to Barneys—and lust over the Prada shoes and the Versace. Now I could almost afford these things. I bought my first pair of Prada shoes, these square-toe slip-on loafers, while I was still in school. I bought a charcoal-gray Versace T-shirt with black cap sleeves and a textured nylon material running down the back. In retrospect, it was hideous, and I wore it all the time. I bought a black Alexander McQueen knit polo with this viscose material weaved through it. I still remember the tag, which was black with red lettering. It felt luxurious. We wore street clothing to work, and I was into tight tops and Versace jeans and Miu Miu shoes. We always turned it out for Saturday nights, when the regular customers came in. Our look was definitely late-nineties Toronto gay—Euro and super-tight.

> "I was working with a bunch of lost souls. But they were lost souls I loved being around. Every night there felt like a performance."

I was out all the time, dancing after work, doing drugs with friends and coworkers. But wasn't everyone? This was college. This is what being twenty years old in a big city for the first time is all about. At least that's what I thought. I didn't yet recognize that I had a problem. Because an addict doesn't see it coming. That's why people stay using. That's why people die. It's because they can't see the signs.

Still, I knew enough to hide it all from Trish Lahde, a classmate from theater school. Trish was from Sault Ste. Marie in Northern Ontario, a place even farther removed than Port Perry. The winters at theater school were long, the days even longer, and we often emerged from the bowels of the refrigeration and upholstery classrooms in the dark. But we had each other. With Trish, I was clean. With Trish I was Bradley Goreski from Port

Perry. We watched teen comedies from the eighties together and danced to Madonna. One night, I showed her videos from elementary school. She started to cry.

Despite my best efforts, the abuse was not helping my performance in school. I was exhausted all the time. Luckily this was theater school and the curriculum was full of exercises where one was asked to lie down on the ground and act like animals. There were days where we pretended to be in "zones of silence." One day, I actually fell asleep on the floor, and the teacher called me out on it, really ripping into me. I swiftly jumped in, explaining, "I have chronic fatigue syndrome. I can't really help it. It's not my fault." I don't know where the lie came from. I guess I was better at improvisation than I thought. And the teacher was convinced. Not only did he believe my excuse, but in my year-end progress report, he praised me for my perseverance. "Despite his chronic fatigue syndrome," he wrote, "Brad is still able to succeed."

But six months later, I couldn't really hide the addiction anymore. I was working at the restaurant, staying out all night, and then trying to go to class. I couldn't see how far out of balance I was. I thought I was holding it together. Addicts always do. But others knew. My parents made the hour-long drive into Toronto every Sunday night to take me grocery

> "I thought I was holding it together. Addicts always do. But others knew."

shopping. Back then, I just thought they wanted to spend time with me. Later I realized that wasn't it at all. They took me grocery shopping because they didn't want to give me the cash. Because they knew what I'd spend it on.

Soon, the school administration asked me to leave. I pushed back and was put on probation instead. It felt like a terrible rejection. Theater school can be a test of self-esteem; you open old wounds in class to find a character, and to have my weaknesses thrown back at me felt like too

"And I learned a valuable lesson that year: You can't let someone take your dream away from you."

much. I dug in my heels. I refused to be a failure. I was stubborn, like a Leo. School was something I wanted. And I learned a valuable lesson that year: You can't let someone take your dream away from you. My teachers rejected me, but they couldn't deny my success in a play called *Dancock's Dance* by Guy Vanderhaeghe. I portrayed a schizophrenic man-child in an asylum, a kid who believes he is the king

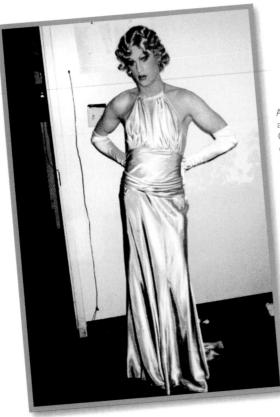

As a theater student at George Brown College in Toronto, I dressed as Marlene Dietrich for a cabaret show, singing "Mean to Me" live. My teachers believed this undercut my talent and that I'd embarrassed myself.

of Germany and is sexually abused by the other patients, and there wasn't a dry eye in the theater.

Sometimes it was all too much. One afternoon early in the third year of drama school, I stood outside one of our classrooms, crying hysterically into my hands, collapsing onto Trish's shoulder. She was my touchstone. But as much as I tried to hide my drug use from her, she knew it was more than recreational.

"I need help," I said. "I need help. I can't do this anymore."

Trish was holding me. She was the nonjudgmental voice of reason. "Whatever you need," she said. "Do you want to leave? Do you need to go home?"

I went to exactly one Cocaine Anonymous meeting, but it didn't take. I wasn't ready. I couldn't yet see that everything was connected. I hadn't hit rock bottom. I still had a roof over my head. I was still holding down a job. I was still functioning. A few weeks later Trish asked me about the meeting, but I dismissed her, telling her I felt nothing. And when she tried to ask me again a few weeks later, I blew her off. I turned a deaf ear to the voice of reason.

The only voice I heard now belonged to a man. A gorgeous man named Nick.

Graduation was approaching, and I was out one night with a drag queen named Tiger Lily, a Pocahontas look-alike with curly black hair (her own). We were way up above the dance floor looking down at a sea of shirtless men. And there was Nick, dressed in jeans and nothing else, his eyes closed, moving to the music.

"If I could date anyone in Toronto," I told Tiger Lily, "it would be him."

A few months later, in March of 1999, she and I were at the Snowflake Ball—or some other party where cardboard snowflakes hang from the ceiling—and there was Nick again. Except this time he was walking directly toward me. I was twenty-one years old. He was forty-three and told me he had two children. It wasn't the kind of news one expects to hear at a club where grown men are sucking on Ring Pops and wearing angel wings. But there we were.

It felt like a scene out of a movie. I was this skinny kid with a bad Caesar haircut and semi-bad clothes, hanging out with low-rent drag queens and people who weren't all that cool. I was always on the outside looking in. I still felt like that kid on *Electric Circus,* the one who was asked to dance in the window hidden behind a sheet. And then Nick showed up. And he was so handsome—like a cross between George Clooney and the guy from *General Hospital,* the one who plays Sonny. And he was talking to me! And I could feel so many pairs of eyes on me, wondering who I was, wondering why this man who everyone wanted was suddenly interested in me. I felt like an ugly duckling finally becoming a swan. I felt a sense of self-worth for the first time. And that night, we closed the place down.

"It felt like a scene out of a movie."

Four months later I moved into Nick's house, not quite in the suburbs, but not quite in the city either. I was domestic. And I was trying to be clean. While it sounds like a bad made-for-Logo movie, I have to say, the relationship started out well enough. Actually, it was kind of like that movie *Stepmom,* right down to the scene where Nick's daughter and I danced in her room doing her hair. I gave her style tips, too. I took her out to lunch.

And ours was this thrilling Gay-December relationship. He was the first man to take me on a proper date. We went to restaurants I'd passed by in the gay area of Toronto and only dreamed of going into. Places I used to walk by and think, I can't even afford to buy a drink there. But suddenly I was inside having an appetizer *and* dinner. I was used to eating the eight-dollar bowl of stir-fry from a place called Spring Rolls, and now I was one of the pretty people.

It was very romantic. I was still working at the restaurant, and I'd get off the late shift and go meet Nick and his friends somewhere to dance. He was friends with *the* group in Toronto. The muscle boys. The cool go-go dancers. The cool lesbian couples. When I'd go out with them, I was so skinny I looked like a Chihuahua in a room full of pit bulls. I was this wispy thing with my little fashions. I'd go into Nick's closet and style him for the night. He didn't care about fashion but he loved Madonna and he loved me and it was heaven. I'd been obsessed with Gianni Versace, and a few years earlier when his boyfriend murdered him, I'd had a meltdown for a couple of days. And

> "Ours was this thrilling Gay-December relationship."

so, when Nick and I went to Florida for New Year's Eve 1999 to celebrate the millennium, my first stop was the Versace mansion to pay my respects. That night, Nick and I dressed in matching silver pants (made out of plastic!) with tight white T-shirts and black shoes and silver bandannas around our necks. Did I regret this look? No way. Who regrets wearing anything in Miami? I was fake-tanned and ready to go—there's no other way to survive the Toronto winter. (I do, however, regret the time in college when I fell asleep in the tanning bed and the manager didn't wake me up. I was in there for fifteen minutes and couldn't participate in my classes for two days because I was so badly charred and couldn't lay down on my back. You could actually see the imprint of where the lightbulbs had been. It was not cute.)

Life with Nick was a whirlwind: I was dancing to Deborah Cox remixes and Whitney Houston was making a comeback and I knew all the lyrics and it was always five in the morning and we were shutting down some club and going to the twenty-four-hour deli to get ice cream and Gummi bears. We'd stay awake until the sun came up and we'd talk and laugh and then the next weekend we'd do it all again. Nick came into my life at a time when my parents were divorcing. My mother had called me over Thanksgiving to ask if I was coming home. I was, I said, and she answered, "Good. It'll be the last Thanksgiving we spend together as a family." In that time, Nick was so gentle. He'd been through a divorce himself and he knew the effect it could have on someone.

I thought, Maybe life will carry on like this forever. But my lifestyle started to ruin relationships. My sister and I weren't getting along. She was in a serious relationship with her first love and their life together was crumbling, leaving her devastated. She didn't call to tell me. What good would I have been to her? We'd drifted apart, and she knew my drug use was more than recreational. It sounds crazy, but I found out about her breakup in a dream. Our grandmother Ruby had always said that Mandy and I were more like twins than brother and sister. We had that cosmic connection that twins share. As damaged as I was then, I had a dream one night that my sister and her boyfriend were splitting up, and I called her the next morning. "I want to know if you're OK," I said. She wasn't OK. Neither of us were.

> "We'd stay awake until the sun came up and we'd talk and laugh and then the next weekend we'd do it all again."

It was all coming to a head. Tracy, my best friend from high school, was studying at Ryerson University, Toronto's answer to the School of Visual Arts. She was eight subway stops away all of this time but we made excuses about not getting together. When we did see each other, she didn't hide her concerns. Finally, we'd made plans, but when I showed up at her apartment, she was horrified. I was so skinny, and I hadn't slept in days. It was a moment of reckoning. She'd wanted to believe that everything would work out for me. When you are young you can fool yourself into believing anything is possible, despite what you see plainly in front of you. We made awkward conversation and after twenty minutes I left. She couldn't watch me hurt myself. We didn't see each other again for six months.

I needed to get help. It was early on a December morning, and Nick was asleep in the next room. I was in our bathroom, staring in the mirror, and I didn't recognize myself. Finally, I felt the weight of the situation. Finally it was real. I told myself, You can carry on like this and the drugs will be your life. You can accept the fact that you're going to live this life and get by with this restaurant job. Or you can stop all of this and try to fulfill the potential that other people see in you. And have always seen in you. For a minute I fought back. Wait, I thought, this is what young people do! They try to find themselves and they do drugs and they experiment. But actually, I realized, I wasn't doing anything with my life except wasting it.

Nick thought I should get sober, but there was only so much he could do. And only so much he wanted me to do. He liked our life of long dinners and late nights. He said, "You don't need to stop drinking, you just need to stop using cocaine." But it was clear to me: I couldn't get healthy in that house. I couldn't be with Nick if I wanted to be alive to see another Christmas.

I called my dad from a pay phone on a street corner in Toronto in the dead of winter. I was crying in heaving sobs, saying how I needed to get sober, saying that Nick and I were breaking up. And I was fine for another few months, sober even, going to AA meetings and crashing on Tracy's couch. Until I saw Nick out at a club one night making out with someone else. And I fell off the wagon. When you're in AA they tell you, "If you don't understand the teachings of Alcoholics Anonymous, you will when you relapse." And I understood it now. The drugs had stopped working. Nick and I stopped working. And I forced myself back to AA.

It was May 3, 2001. I was determined to stay sober. This was day one: the first day of the rest of my life.

There was the detangling, and it wasn't easy. In April, my father pulled up to Nick's house to help me move out. "It's a hard thing you're doing," my dad said. While he didn't say much else that morning, that was enough.

It was cold out, I remember that. Nick had been giving me the silent treatment, but finally he cracked. "Why would I talk to you!" he shouted. "I have nothing to say to you." As our van pulled away from the curb that David Gray song "Babylon" came on the radio. The lyrics stung:

I've been afraid. To tell you how I really feel, admit to some of those bad mistakes I've made.

"Can we please turn this off?" I said.

It was a turning point. Over the next few months, I attended regular AA meetings in Toronto. I had a new, sober group of friends and I was grateful for them. I made my amends, with my sister first, then with my mother. I was still working at the restaurant, but I decided I was going to leave Toronto. I didn't know when I'd go, and I didn't know where I'd go. But I knew I would leave. That much was certain. And I started preparing for it. I started putting money away—half of my tips each night went into an envelope that I kept hidden behind a broken computer in the bedroom.

I'd finished school only to discover that I didn't want to be an actor. Of the thirty kids in the program at George Brown, only thirteen of us graduated. And I'd landed my first professional acting gig—a gay play put on at Buddies in Bad Times, a well-respected regional theater known for shock value. I quickly realized I didn't have the drive to be a successful actor, and that was OK. I'd tried it on for size and it didn't fit.

> **"I was in our bathroom, staring in the mirror, and I didn't recognize myself."**

Something else soon came up—an unlikely career option but maybe a fine escape route. I was out one night when a man approached me and suggested I try modeling. OK, truth time: I was flattered. But I knew what I looked like. I was cute. I took cute pictures. But I wasn't a *male model*. Especially not with that bad haircut. I wasn't quite tall enough, either.

Breaking Up Is Hard to Do

A PLAYLIST TO MEND A BROKEN HEART

"Unbreak My Heart," Toni Braxton

"Here with Me," Dido

"Stronger," Britney Spears

"Fear," Sarah McLachlan

"Someone Like You," Adele

"Try Sleeping with a Broken Heart," Alicia Keys

"Nobody's Supposed to Be Here," Deborah Cox

"Bleeding Love," Leona Lewis

"Call Your Girlfriend," Robyn

"It's Not Right but It's Okay," Whitney Houston

"No More Drama," Mary J. Blige

"Tralala," Lush

"Get Outta My Way," Kylie Minogue

"Find Your Love," Drake

"Single Ladies (Put a Ring on It)," Beyoncé

But I was looking for a parachute out of Toronto, and maybe this was it. The next day, I walked into the Ford Modeling Agency, and while they liked my cheekbones, I was a hair too short for runway work. Thankfully, a lesser (but still reputable) firm, Armstrong Model Agency, took me on. I was still not invited to the party! I was a "male model," but I wasn't at the best agency. I landed work, and yet I was in a Dentyne chewing gum commercial—with my back to the camera. I posed for the Sears catalog in khakis, which were all the wrong size for me. It was exciting, though I didn't know how the shoot was supposed to work. "What's going on?" I asked. The photographer said, "We're taking product shots."

"Cool," I said. Until I realized that "product shots" meant you'd never see my face. Oh, well.

I soon met a representative from a Greek modeling agency who said if I could get myself to Greece for the summer, he'd represent me. And I took it. It was an emotional moment. My mom and sister were devastated to see me go. I'd had long, up-all-night conversations with my mom about what I was going to do with my life and how I needed to get out of the rut I was in. At the airport, she refused to cry. She knew this was the right thing for me. And she didn't want me to see her break. She didn't want me to see how much pain she was in.

I was supposed to be in Greece for two months. I had $1,500 in my pocket and the lessons of AA running through my head. One day at a time. Easy does it.

My life in Athens might not have been glamorous, but it was a wild adventure and exactly what I needed. I pulled up to my new home and the sign read HOTEL TONY. If there was an actual Tony, I never met him. There was no view of the Aegean Sea, just twin beds for the bargain price of four thousand drachmas a night—or less than twenty American dollars. I was sharing the room with Francesco, a male model from Portugal who didn't speak English but was very hot. I pointed at objects in the room and said, "bed" and "clo-set," while he tried to sound out the words. I quickly made friends with Esther, a model from London, and we traveled around together. It was amazing.

I was expected to get work immediately. Unfortunately, at the precise time I arrived in Greece to make my modeling debut, the fashion world took a sharp turn. Tastes changed and all of the designers wanted buff male models with long hair. My look—close-cropped hair, bony frame, preppy style—was out. Yet there I was, toting my modeling portfolio

"I wasn't booking jobs, but I certainly felt glamorous."

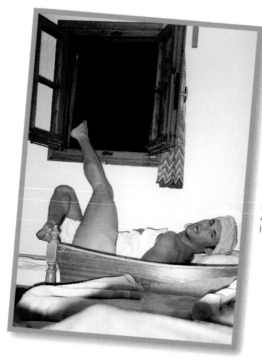

At a hotel in Mykonos. I was dancing to "The Boss" by Diana Ross—my favorite Diana Ross song. As for the turban? It's a look.

around Athens. I went on plenty of modeling appointments but I didn't book any modeling jobs.

I wasn't complaining, believe me. It's not like I was working in a salt mine or anything. I wasn't booking jobs, but I certainly felt glamorous. Forget the Toronto club scene. I was running around Athens with a pack of models. And the local club owners were so desperate to have a fashionable crowd adorn their places that they invited us in for free. This was the island of misfit, handsome toys. I didn't really belong with this crowd; I knew that. But I'd rather have been there at the beach staring out at the most beautiful crystal-blue water than just about anywhere else in the world.

I was broke in Greece, but I didn't care. We ate souvlaki and smoked cigarettes all night. I met a Greek guy from Canada who showed me around town and acted as my translator. I met a gay ex-military Greek guy who became obsessed with me. I decided to take a weeklong vacation to Mykonos. What I needed a vacation from, who knows? But I booked a dirt-cheap motel for seven drachmas a night. I was going only for a week, but this Greek soldier followed me to the airport and took a photograph of my plane taking off. It was a true Greek tragedy.

There was a moment of reckoning. What was I doing in Greece? Was I just running away, or was something more profound going on? Yes, I'd always wanted to see Greece. I'd had a friend in Toronto named Markos who was Greek and talked nonstop about how beautiful it was there. (Side note: His mother would cry every time we went out dancing. "Why are you going out so late?" She also refused to acknowledge that her son was gay— even though he wore red sequin-and-rhinestone cowboy boots.) But it was more than that. Something Nick said came back to me. We'd had a fight about my relationship with my mother. About how I called her too often,

Boardwalk Empire

SIX ESSENTIALS FOR A DAY AT THE BEACH

1. Flip-flops are meant for the sand. But not for anywhere else.
2. Your bathing suit is not an outfit. The beach is a big, sandy runway—even for men. Wear a button-up shirt or a polo. Wear a boat shoe on the beach, or a driving loafer. Wear a flip-flop to dress down an outfit. Get it together.
3. A cute beach bag is a must. And it doesn't have to be expensive. A cute $10 tote from H&M will do.
4. Beach towels: They don't have to be Hermès, but please, no frayed edges.
5. Bring a book. Even if you're not going to read it.
6. Don't just sit there and text on your phone. It's gross. Engage with your surroundings. You're at the beach. Look up!

about how I was needy. Though I didn't realize it at the time, Nick wasn't really talking about my mom. He was telling me that I needed to grow up. And there I was, clean and sober, living on my own in a foreign country, proving to myself that I could do something. *That's* what modeling was about for me.

When I first landed in Greece, I'd made a pact with myself. My world at home in Toronto had become so small, this insular cave of drugs and alcohol. Now I was turning a corner. I would be open to new experiences. I would see what cards the world dealt me. I would let chance play out. I would live again. I would be naïve again. I didn't want anything to tie me down. I didn't get sober to be miserable.

The best-laid plans of male models . . .

I was on vacation in Mykonos with my friend Tony, the Canadian Greek translator. It was July and hot as hell, but the sea felt like a silk Hermès scarf on my neck. We were walking down the main thoroughfare, in a stream of people, like salmon swimming downstream, when we passed a restaurant called Nico's Taverna. Outside, my translator recognized his friend Sal, who was sitting having dinner with another friend. And they flagged us down.

While Tony and Sal were catching up, they left me and Sal's friend Gary Janetti—an American—idling there awkwardly. I was dressed in what Gary would later describe as "Eurotrash jeans." Which had something to do with the excessive amounts of contrast stitching on the acid-wash denim. I was also wearing a blue T-shirt, and I still had that Caesar haircut. I am proud of none of this today, but I am trying to paint the picture. If I acted aloof at first, it was only because I was trying to be a free spirit. I'd been broken up with my boyfriend for two months. But as soon as Gary offered me a bite of his dessert, I melted. He started to tell me about his life in Los Angeles. He wrote for television, he said, but he'd grown up in New York. I told him about Canada, about how I was obsessed with the tenth-anniversary concert of *Les Misérables* starring Patti LuPone, which had been airing on Canadian public television before I left. (This is the kind of shit I used to tape on the VHS; when I was a kid, I'd record the Tony Awards and watch the ceremony over and over again. Likewise with the red carpet at the Oscars.) Gary talked about his nieces and how they'd just visited and were listening to this song "Survivor" by Destiny's Child over and over again. We'd been making idle chitchat for hours when he asked me if I wanted to go dancing. We were out until three in the morning.

I was supposed to go back to Athens in the morning—modeling appointments awaited. Instead, I hopped a plane to Santorini with Gary and Sal. And over the course of a week, Gary and I got to know each other. I was impressed with his resolve. He grew up in Queens and not too long ago had been a frustrated writer working as a bellhop at a New York hotel. Until he up and quit, moved to Los Angeles, and landed a job writing for a major network series in less than a year. He saw huge potential in himself, saw that a transformation was possible, and acted on it. It was the first example I'd seen of someone taking such a risk, and I was drawn to him as a source of inspiration. It's not very Canadian to change courses so radically. But Gary had done it, and wonderfully so. Could I do the same?

> "While it may sound cliché, I felt something different with Gary. He saw something in me that I thought was lost."

On the beach in Santorini, Gary and I were talking about seeing each other again, at first half-joking, and then more directly. He knew I was a huge Madonna fan. She was scheduled to perform in L.A. later that summer. "Come for a visit," Gary said. "We'll see Madonna. And we'll see what this is."

I wasn't sure how to respond. It's easy to fall in love when you are in Greece. But it is something else to take that love to the mainland. And yet,

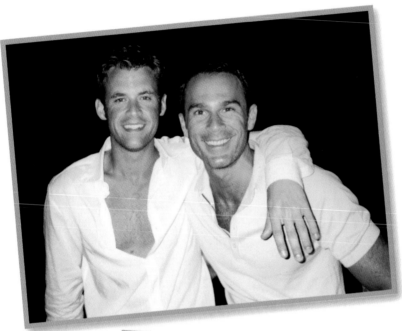

Gary and me,
Greece, 2001.

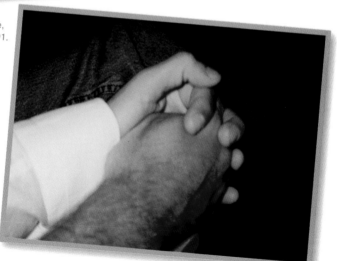

while it may sound cliché, I felt something different with Gary. He saw something in me that I thought was lost. I had a flashback to kindergarten and my teacher Mrs. Chandler telling my mom that I was going to be fine. That I had a spark she needed to nurture, not beat down. In the years since—especially during college—I'd convinced myself that the spark had burned out for good. But Gary saw it flickering, however faint. Despite my patchwork jeans that flared out, despite the bad vintage T-shirt I was wearing, which was the height of gay Canadian fashion—despite all of that he saw something in this kid from Ontario who'd never been to New York, who had been a waiter yet had somehow made his way to Greece, who carried a Prada messenger bag and was obsessed with musical theater.

We kissed good-bye and he went off to the airport. He told me to call him when I was ready to come visit him in Los Angeles. Whenever that is, he said, I'll be waiting.

He didn't have to wait very long. By the time Gary landed in L.A. there was a message waiting for him at home. "I want to come visit," I said. "I'm ready." Surely there is more to life than this hotel in Greece, I thought. There must be. But what is next? Where am I going?

It is time to look.

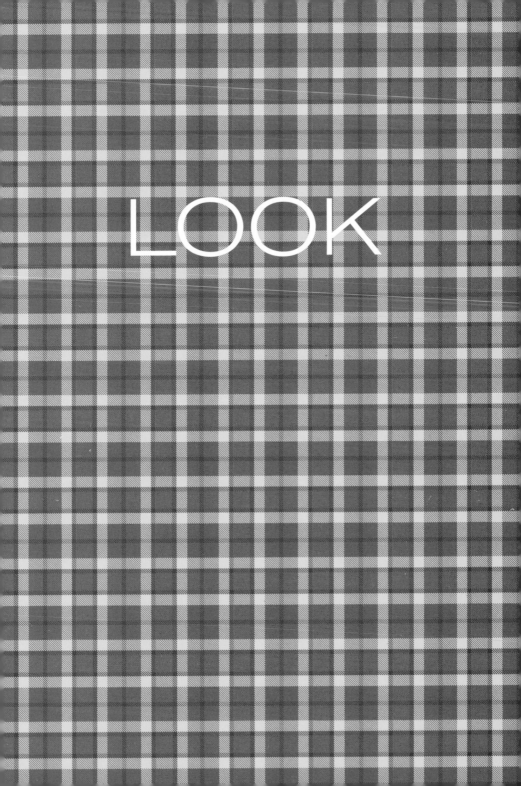

LOOK

4

New York is waiting for you.
And it's not only for the rich.

ASK GARY ABOUT MY arrival in Los Angeles, and he will tell you that the first thing out of my mouth wasn't "hello" or "Thank you for the plane ticket," but rather these words: "They lost my luggage." In my defense, I'd brought my best clothing with me to Athens and that lost suitcase was full of Miu Miu shoes, Prada, Versace, Alexander McQueen, and anything else in my wardrobe worth owning. It was a couple of years' worth of shopping and I could never afford to buy it all back, and now it was on some sad baggage carousel in South America or somewhere going round and round.

And here we were: two relative strangers playing house.

I took to L.A. very quickly. I got Balinese highlights, the kind of treatment where the pigment is brushed onto your hair so it looks sun kissed. I wanted to look like Brad Pitt in *Ocean's Eleven*. As promised, we went to the Madonna concert, with Gary calling in a favor from, of all people, Gwyneth Paltrow's assistant. We were in the tenth row of a sold-out show. I wore my olive Gucci dress shirt and by the time the night was over, my hair was standing straight up. Someone behind me must have eaten a pretzel, because I had mustard all over my back. I was sweating through everything on my body. Gary took one look at me and said, "What happened to you?"

> "And here we were: two relative strangers playing house."

"I had an out-of-body experience," I said.

Which was sort of how I felt in L.A. I wondered, What am I going to do with my life? For a minute, I thought maybe I'd try modeling again. I knew I didn't really have what it takes, but I found out when the modeling agencies had their open calls, and I toted my portfolio all over town. No one bit. I didn't have a green card, so I couldn't really get a job. And so I took hip-hop classes. I got my driver's license.

And I used the time to get to know Gary. It was a period of great exploration, a chance for us to build a real foundation. It was a time of many firsts. My first trip to London. My first trip to Thailand. I was very into this idea of American sportiness. I wore slogan T-shirts from Urban Outfitters. I wore nostalgic, faded Mickey Mouse decals. I spent too many afternoons driving up and down Melrose looking for the perfect vintage T-shirts for Gary and me. I wore cargo pants with novelty T-shirts and a Gucci monogrammed hat with Nike Shocks. It was almost the reverse of drag, and a very early-2000s moment.

I also made my first trip to New York City. Gary grew up in Queens, and shortly after the Twin Towers fell, he became desperate to take me home. "You're never going to see the city I grew up in," he said. But he felt strongly that we should infuse some cash into the tourist-strapped city. And so we landed at JFK and took a car into Manhattan, and when the skyline came into view for the first time my heart beat out of my chest. It was exactly as I imagined it would be. SoHo. Fifth Avenue. *The Music Man*! Within a few days, I was riding the subway by myself like it had always been this way. Manhattan and I were in love.

While I was happy in Los Angeles, my family had their suspicions. Moving to L.A. with a man I barely knew? It had a faint whiff of Nick, like there was some gay-jà vu happening. My sister was indignant. When I called to explain she actually said, "This is crap." For months now she had been at home in Canada stewing, refusing to support this plan. Finally, Gary confronted the situation head-on, picking up the phone and offering to fly her to Los Angeles so they could meet face-to-face, which she did. Tracy, my high school friend whom I styled for the prom, was similarly concerned. "You don't know this person," she said. "You're taking an enormous leap of faith." She actually ended her rant with these words: "Here we go again." While she was a struggling young professional in Toronto, she was so concerned that she put a wildly expensive plane ticket on her credit card and flew to L.A. so she could conduct her due diligence.

> "When the skyline came into view for the first time my heart beat out of my chest."

And she was relieved to find that Gary was as good as I described. I took Tracy around town. We went to the beach in Malibu and ran around on the sand and took pictures of each other. Unfortunately, our outfits were fashion don'ts. I was wearing a jean vest. It reminds me of how we used to be in high school—doing silly photo shoots and wearing clothes that we thought were cool at the time but that we'd regret in six months. I took her to Palm Springs and we sat at the diner and ordered burgers and fries and Oreo milkshakes. We went to a gay bar but spent more time sitting on the curb outside the 7-Eleven across the street, drinking Red

Bull and gossiping. Sitting outside a convenience store is a very Canadian thing to do. You can take the boy out of Ontario but you can't take Ontario out of the boy. Swept up in the glamour of Los Angeles, Tracy bought a Marc Jacobs jacket at Fred Segal that she couldn't afford and a Vuitton purse on Rodeo Drive just because. That night, with our feet in the backyard swimming pool at Gary's house, Tracy cried. It wasn't buyer's remorse. Nothing like that. Rather, she was crying from contentment. Because when she looked in my eyes, she once again saw her old friend from Port Perry. She could once again feel the spirit of kinship between us, between two like-minded souls who'd met on the first day of high school—me in the color-block Polo rugby, she in all-black Le Château—and dreamed of something more. We had drifted apart, but we were back together. And we'd figure the next steps out, just like we did as teenagers.

She was struggling in her own life and was contemplating a move to New York. "How do I do it?" she said.

"Pack up a U-Haul and drive across the border," I said. "You'll get a job. You'll figure it out."

I didn't have any great wisdom—just enough sense to know that if she wanted something badly enough, she would figure it out. Because that's what I was doing every day.

I was finding my way in Los Angeles. After a few months, I joined a well-known Alcoholics Anonymous outpost in Brentwood. This was no touchy-feely L.A. support group. Here, they didn't coddle their members. They didn't care if your car broke down and you couldn't make the meeting. There were no excuses. No matter what, you made the meeting. You checked in. It was tough love. No one cared about your problems. No one cared that you broke a nail and it made you want to drink. There were people in the group whose children were killed by drunk drivers. All they cared about was that you maintained your sobriety. If you were so miserable and you wanted to wallow in that misery, go have a drink. We were there to get well. We were there to live life.

That is what I wanted. Los Angeles could be a lonely place, and I counted on Gary for all of my entertainment, which put a strain on the still-new relationship. He was happy for us to have the time together. But he was adamant that I have my own experiences. For a relationship to work, he said, two people need to learn from each other. And he was right. He wanted me to blaze my own trail. When you are lost, it is too easy to give yourself up to somebody else. He wanted me to find what I was looking for. To survive, he said, I'd need to create a life for myself. The thought resonated. One of the tenets of AA is that to propel yourself forward, you need to stop taking from other people. On so many levels I had to create something for myself.

And so, just as suddenly, I was a twenty-four-year-old freshman at Santa Monica College, hoping to earn enough credits to transfer to USC. I was waiting for a sign, waiting to figure out what

> "For a relationship to work, he said, two people need to learn from each other."

was next for me. Until then, I would drive myself to school at five thirty in the morning, because I preferred to go to the cafeteria and get work done than sit in rush-hour traffic. I was enrolled in general education classes, taking the lowest level of math. I took yoga classes and art history classes and journalism. I bought new spiral notebooks and new pens and pencils. The scene at school reminded me of *Clueless,* when Alicia Silverstone gives Brittany Murphy a tour around campus, explaining to her about the different cliques. We, too, had burnouts on the grassy knoll. We also had kids who hoped to transfer to bigger schools. We had wealthy kids in Range Rovers and head-to-toe Gucci and full makeup and blown-out hair. It was this great cross-section. I hung out with the Japanese exchange students. They have amazing style and they love fashion. They gave me exotic Japanese candies and I returned the favor by helping them with their English, and we exchanged stories of our cultures. I took French. In a prescient sign of the future to come, Guinevere van Seenus

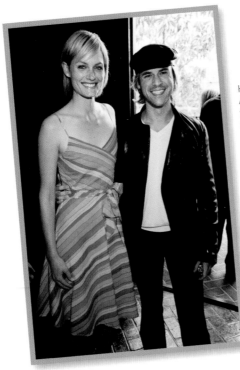

Here I am posing with model Amber Valletta at a benefit for the Friendly House in Los Angeles. This photo has surfaced before, and people often use it as a chance to say, "Brad Goreski wasn't always so stylish!" But I disagree. This hat? It's leather and it's Tom Ford for Gucci. And it's amazing. And it hides the fact that I had a blow-out for this party.

sat in front of me in class. I told her she should be a model. She smiled politely. When I went home and googled her, I found out she'd been on the cover of Italian *Vogue* at least twice. Uh-oh.

The joke of being a twenty-four-year-old college freshman was not lost on me. But I refused to take this lightly. I felt I had been given a second chance at life, and I didn't want to waste it. And for the first time in my life my eyes were wide open. I vowed to learn the importance of looking at one's surroundings. Of taking notes. Of observing. But what was I going to do with my life? Where was I going?

Gary and I were sitting on the couch one afternoon, and I was flipping through *V* magazine, talking about the photo shoots I loved and why the styling was so perfect. "You're always talking about clothes and reading fashion magazines and looking at what people are wearing," Gary said. "Why not do something in fashion?"

It was like the heavens parting. It's odd that I didn't think of fashion myself. But looking back, it just seemed too far away, too impossible. How would I get there? How would I break into one of the hardest industries in the world? How would I take the first step when I could see only how far away the goal was?

> **"I felt I had been given a second chance at life, and I didn't want to waste it. And for the first time in my life my eyes were wide open."**

But now I knew this was what I needed to do. Looking back, my childhood was all about listening to my heart. And this is when I heard it again: the voice of Barbie calling me. I saw an eleven-year-old, overweight Brad Goreski in front of the television watching Jeanne Beker interview Marc Jacobs on Canadian TV, talking about his grunge collection for Perry Ellis. *This* was what I loved. Fashion was my calling.

had opened myself up to the possibilities of a new life. This new life started with my telling anyone who would listen that I was looking for a job in fashion. I was sent an unlikely guardian angel in the form of Sara Switzer, an editor at *Vanity Fair,* who also happened to be Sandra Bernhard's girlfriend. I was—and am still—obsessed with Sandra's show *Without You I'm Nothing.* Gary and I were at a dinner

> **"*This* was what I loved. Fashion was my calling."**

party, and I was introduced to Sara. She was asking me all kinds of questions about what I was studying at school and what I wanted to do later. She took a vested interest in me and my future. I told her that a dream of mine was to intern at *Vogue.* Lo and behold, Michelle Sanders,

Rent This Movie!

WITHOUT YOU I'M NOTHING (1990)

When I was working at Five Doors North, my coworker James lent me his VHS copy of Sandra Bernhard's smash-hit one-woman show from 1987, *Without You I'm Nothing*. Of course I knew who she was, but I had never seen her perform. I was instantly obsessed. Sandra incorporates humor, social commentary, politics, pop culture, sexuality, fashion, pathos, and song into her performance. (Memorable quote: "My father's a proctologist. My mother's an abstract artist. That's how I view the world.") She has created her own form of theater that is completely faithful to her point of view and the way she sees the world. I've seen her perform many times and it is always a unique, wildly entertaining, and intelligent night. I adore her. If you have not seen her perform, do yourself a favor and go!

the accessories editor at *Vogue,* was a good friend of hers, and Sara said she'd be happy to help me get an interview. She was simply being kind, I know that. But in her kindness was grace. I wasn't sure if she understood the impact her introduction and faith had on my life, but it was significant, sending me off on a wild ride. I am still grateful to her for that kind gesture.

It happened quicker than I could have possibly imagined. There was no conference call with the human resources department at Condé Nast, the parent company of *Vogue* (and countless other luxury magazines). All it took was a phone call to the accessories editor, and after my freshman year at Santa Monica College I was on my way to New York for a summer internship at the very magazine I used to smuggle up to my bedroom.

I deplaned at JFK airport and climbed into a yellow taxicab, the Manhattan skyline once again coming into view. It appeared different this time, perhaps because I was not on vacation. This time, I would be a New Yorker. And I was instantly enlivened, as if the spirit of a Danceteria-era Madonna herself rushed through my veins. I felt this was the Manhattan of *Guys and Dolls* and *Fame* and *Annie*. This was the place where Stephen Sprouse and Keith Haring and Basquiat and Peter Lindbergh first made their marks, a place for artists and designers to come for inspiration. It all seemed so dangerous. I had dreamed of this moment for years, down to the smell of the cupcakes from Magnolia Bakery, which was just down the street from the apartment. I didn't dream of late-night parties or the nightlife. I dreamed of something more ephemeral, of walking out my front door every day and being confronted by Manhattan. I dreamed of double-fisting Magnolia's banana pudding and the yellow cake with the buttercream icing all at once.

At twenty-four years of age, I was the oldest summer intern in Anna Wintour's kingdom. And I was deadly serious about the job. I was living in a one-bedroom sublet on Charles Street; Gary's friend James, a writer, was away in Provincetown for the summer and agreed to sublet the rent-stabilized apartment to me for the bargain-basement price of $1,200. Like all New York apartments, this one had its quirks—namely, an elderly neighbor who slammed her front door every time she came and went, so much so that the dishes and glassware in James's apartment rattled. We came to call her "Donna Door Slammer." But trust me, this place was a steal. Not least of all because it was in the West Village, around the corner from 66 Perry Street, an address made famous by *Sex and the City*. (While Carrie Bradshaw lived on the Upper East Side, the actual front stoop where they shot is on Perry.)

> "I dreamed of double-fisting Magnolia's banana pudding and the yellow cake with the buttercream icing all at once."

This sounds crazy in retrospect, but I can't remember what I wore on my first day of work. But I know how I felt emerging from the elevator on the twelfth floor of the Condé Nast Building in Times Square. And what I felt in my bones was that I'd absolutely 100 percent worn the wrong thing. Over the next eight weeks of this sometimes-glamorous internship, there would be many days where I felt this way. It was too late. Like all new interns, I gave my name to the security guard in the lobby and he sent me on my way. The thought going through my head was simple: How did I get here?

In the twelfth-floor lobby I was greeted by the manager of the accessories closet—located across the hall from the fashion closet—and after the briefest of office tours I was deposited in our cramped, windowless space. There were four desks around the perimeter of the accessories closet, plus a wall of the latest handbags and Manolos kept under lock and key. But most of the action took place around a center island, a mess of drawers with tissue paper on top. This was where we stored all of the jewelry for the upcoming *Vogue* photo shoots. Millions of dollars in gold and baubles passed through that room every day. In the accessories closet, we, the overwashed masses of interns, huddled around the island and cataloged the pieces that came in, taking Polaroids of the jewels on fresh tissue paper and then immediately packing them back up so they would be ready to go out on a shoot.

No one at *Vogue* told me any of this, by the way. We were taught not to ask questions. What little I knew about my job responsibilities came from the other interns. It was a high-pressure office; that much I understood. Do you know that scene in *The Devil Wears Prada* where Meryl Streep arrives early to the office and the editors scramble around trying to put themselves together before she shows up? That really happens. I know this because one day early that summer a girl wearing denim and unimpressive heels was unexpectedly called into Anna Wintour's office. I've never seen someone give themselves a makeover so quickly. In five minutes, this girl had gone into the fashion closet and changed into a dress, grabbed a pair of Manolos, and put on a full face. I thought, *Vogue* really *is* a magical place.

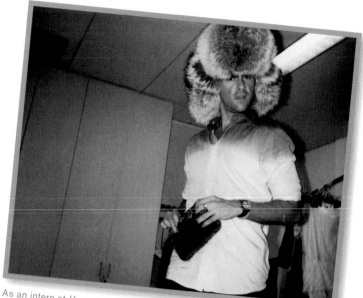

As an intern at *Vogue*. I worked in the accessories closet and never needed a reason to try on a Dior fur hat. There's now a no-try-on rule for interns, and if you're caught messing around you can be fired. Thankfully, that rule wasn't in place in 2004.

From the outside, the environment was pretty—all fresh-cut flowers and scrubbed-clean faces. But underneath it could be a minefield. We had thirty minutes to eat, and we barely took that. You certainly didn't bring food back up to your desk. You weren't checking in jewelry while eating a Cobb salad. I learned very quickly that we interns had to compete among one another like the kids in *The Hunger Games*. We were all angling for the same prize: the chance to go on a real *Vogue* photo shoot. That was the golden ticket. That was our raison d'être. But how to get there? I didn't know how to act. And so I acted like someone from the movies. I acted like I imagined someone who has an apartment in the West Village and an internship at Condé Nast should

> "Vogue really *is* a magical place."

act. I was impossibly serious at all times. I was asleep by eleven. I went to Broadway shows. I went to bookstores and art galleries. I acted like my idea of a Manhattan grown-up.

If every day there felt like a test—and it did—I was desperate to find a study partner. And suddenly there she was. I noticed her shorts first. They were Libertine—*the* downtown label of the moment—and I was endlessly impressed. Even though Libertine shorts were basically chinos purchased at the Goodwill, washed a million times, and then silk-screened with, like, a picture of an eyeball and sold for $900, they were very hip. The girl wearing them interned in the fashion closet, and we met one morning when she wheeled a rack of clothing into the accessories closet.

> "I was asleep by eleven. I went to Broadway shows. I went to bookstores and art galleries. I acted like my idea of a Manhattan grown-up."

"I like your shorts," I said.

"Thanks," she said. "They're my mom's."

Whose mom wears Libertine? I needed to know this girl.

Her name was Danielle Nachmani. Years later she would become a major fashion stylist in New York. But back then she was just the girl with long brown hair and caramel skin and shorts she stole from her mother's closet. Her look was Parisian, in a way; Danielle did menswear but with a feminine touch. She'd wear a men's sweater but with a bra strap showing. She'd wear trousers but with a super-high heel. She wore certain labels not just because they were cute, but because she knew the editors at *Vogue* would notice. That's one way to get ahead. We made fun of the proportions of her oversize JNCO—Judge None, Choose One—pants. Well, I judged! Danielle was wearing super-wide-leg Tsubi jeans one day and I made fun of her because, to me anyway, they looked like jeans that ravers wore in Toronto. All that was missing was a neon plastic chain hanging from her waist and a pacifier around her neck. It turned out that Danielle proved

Closet Case

NINE THINGS EVERY WOMAN NEEDS IN HER WARDROBE

1. A well-tailored blazer

The right blazer—in navy or black—is what we call a fix-all. If you're cold and you need to throw something over your shoulders, this will do. If you can't think about putting an outfit together, you can always grab your perfect blazer, skinny jeans, a pair of cute pumps, and a necklace and you're good to go. A well-tailored blazer is easily woven into all elements of dressing, day or night. The key is that it needs to fit well. Put time into finding the right one. On the affordable end, J.Crew makes a good blazer. Or try Tibi. On the high end, Band of Outsiders and Boy both make great blazers.

2. A party pump

This is the shoe that takes the blazer and jeans from the office into an evening look. The right party pump is something people will talk about. Investing in shoes is important, not necessarily because some inexpensive shoes tend to fall apart, but because the right shoe makes the outfit. Spend $10 on a T-shirt and $30 on a skirt from H&M. Great. But if you have Louboutins on your feet, it elevates the whole outfit. If you're going to collect something in fashion, make it shoes. Pieces come and go seasonally, but shoes are forever. Unless you're buying a super-collection-specific shoe, you can't go wrong. (Even then, you'll save that striped Prada wedge as an archive piece once the season is over.)

3. The little black dress

It's a cliché for a reason. As a topic, how to update the little black dress comes up every few years. But it's not a cliché if you find the right one. Not everyone has the budget to invest in Alaïa or a Dolce

(CONTINUED ON NEXT PAGE)

& Gabbana, and that's fine. The good shoe? The good jewelry? Use that to style up the LBD. How do you know when you've found the right one? You know when you look in the mirror. It's all about the silhouette.

4. The right clutch

What I like about the clutch is that it's a good way to remind yourself that you're about to start a new adventure. If you're going to a nice dinner, even if you're wearing something you wore to the office, you'll add a blazer or change your shoe. Do the same with your bag. No one wants to carry some hefty bag and their iPad to dinner. Put that fun clutch in your day purse and take it out at night. By the way, you need a clutch that actually *holds* things. It doesn't need to be the size of a pill to be cute. You want something functional. And it doesn't need to be Judith Leiber or Prada (though I love those, of course). Just find something small and leather that works for you. If you're outrageous and want to buy something that can be your statement accessory, that works, too. It can be studded, beaded, have feathers on it. Just let it reflect your style.

5. One great pair of jeans

Find the brand that works for you and stick to it. I have probably forty pairs of Levi's in my closet, because they fit me and they're at a great price point. Some of them cost just $49. If you're someone who is into Japanese denim that's never been washed or jeans that were found in the back room of the Levi's archive from the 1970s and only thirty pairs have been made, go for it. Spend $500 on one pair. I support that. As long as it's not boot cut. Cowboys are the only ones who should be wearing boot cut.

6. A really good jewelry set

Think earrings and a ring. Or earrings, a necklace, and a ring. It can even be costume jewelry. You just need a few pieces of statement jewelry you can pepper throughout your looks. It's as simple as having a gold hoop, a gold necklace, and a gold bauble ring. Something easy and eye-catching that doesn't have to break the bank. Check out Alexis Bittar or C. C. Skye. There's great costume jewelry out there; there are even pieces at H&M for $9.99. Find something you love that can update the basics you're wearing to the next level.

7. A great coat

If you live in a cooler climate, you need to invest in a really good winter coat. When you're out in public, your outerwear is what people see half of the year. If you're strapped for cash, wait for the sale and put the coat away for next season. It's worth the investment to find something that reflects who you are. If you see a belted Céline coat on sale for $500, snatch it up. You'll wear it forever.

8. The denim jacket

The right denim jacket is a great layering piece. They look really cute under a trench coat or under a blazer. Whether it's crisp and raw or a worn-in vintage Levi's, they work perfectly over a cocktail dress. Again, it comes down to the fit and the wash. If you like a little DIY, customize it to fit your style. And I should say, I don't mind denim on denim. But I'm Canadian. I could be wrong.

9. The lust item

It's important to have something in your wardrobe that satisfies that luxury desire and need—the one item that you've been lusting after all season. Even if you don't wear it right away. Even if you don't think you'll *ever* wear it, but there's something overpowering you— some voice that says you have to have it. Sometimes just having it in your closet is enough. But the opportunity to wear it will present itself eventually. This is the piece you'll wear that will make everyone freak out. This is how you build fashion self-esteem.

Plus: The Basic Basics

FIVE STAPLES WOMEN CAN'T LIVE WITHOUT

1. Great T-shirts

The neckline is up to you. Some people love a deep V. (I don't.) But every girl should have black, gray, and white at the ready.

2. Functional bras and seamless underwear

A mix of functional and fashionable underwear, including seamless bras. When it comes to underwear, there's nothing worse than a visible panty line. Sometimes it seems like nobody knows that seamless underwear exists. But Calvin Klein makes them. Commando makes them. Hanky Panky makes them. You don't need a drawer full; a few pairs will suffice.

3. Flats

Whether they're Lanvin or they're $19.99 flats from Target, a good pair of flats is a must.

4. The classic white button-up shirt

Or two white shirts, really: one oversize, one tailored. The oversize one is for that eighties Brooke Shields look, which is really modern with denim. It's also great over a bathing suit. You can belt it. You can really do anything with a white shirt. But then there's definitely a place for a tailored white shirt with a navy blazer, white jeans, and a ballet flat. And that place is on the Upper East Side.

5. The right day bag

Whether it's a canvas tote or Givenchy, a day bag you love is essential. It doesn't have to be the fashion It bag of the season, either. Grace Coddington from *Vogue* carries an L.L.Bean tote with her name embroidered on it. No matter what your flavor is, no matter what your style is, you should have a bag that you're happy to carry around every day.

herself to be way more fashion-forward than I was. Because we soon saw Meredith Melling Burke—a stylish editor at *Vogue*—wearing the same pair of Tsubi jeans. Oops! My bad. Not only did I regret making fun of Danielle, but in 2008, when Bottega Veneta started making jeans that were almost identical, I bought two pairs. And I wear them all the time.

Danielle and I talked of nothing but fashion. And we had similar reference points. We both revered this Steven Meisel shoot that *Vogue's* legendary Grace Coddington styled, the one with Kristen McMenamy and Linda Evangelista wearing wispy chiffon Chanel gowns at a French château, based on *The Piano*—with Galliano's collection of unfinished hoop skirts and the shipwrecked Victorian woman with a mass of curls, marooned on a beach surrounded by driftwood.

We were obsessed with models. We were consumed by old Dolce & Gabbana campaigns shot by Steven Meisel. A lot of the interns didn't have the same reference points at their disposal. And some of them didn't even care. Some of those girls just wanted to say they worked at *Vogue*. There was this sense of entitlement that ran through some of them. But Danielle and I didn't have that. We had a strong work ethic and a deep reverence for the magazine as an institution. It was a privilege to be in the hallways of *Vogue*. As an intern, I didn't have any expectations that I'd be hanging out at Anna Wintour's house going over the book every night. I understood that this would be a tough nut to crack and that I should be happy with the position I had—which was the lowest position. (I did see Anna in the elevator once. I almost hit her with my umbrella. I thought, At least the umbrella was Chanel.)

I looked down the line at the other interns one by one and strategically thought, *She's the weak link. She's not into it.* It's not that these girls were rude. Plenty of them were nice girls who lived at the NYU dorm for the summer and liked clothes. But they didn't necessarily *want* it. They didn't want the career. It wasn't so much what they said, but you could tell by what time they left the office. They worked a full day, of course. We all did. But at seven P.M. they might ask their editor if they could go home. They had dinners and appointments with trainers and colonics to get to. But Danielle and I? We didn't have anywhere else to be. And even if we did, we wouldn't have left. At night, people had to tell us to go home. When I worked at the Gap in Toronto I had zero work ethic. But *Vogue*? This was where it was all happening. I worked hard and stayed late because if you left you might miss a miracle. If you left early, you might miss Grace Coddington doing a run-through. You might miss Meredith Melling Burke doing an edit. We were there to learn. And those were the moments that mattered.

I didn't make a dime that summer. I'm not exaggerating. The internship was unpaid, a swap for college credit. It didn't matter. That's one of the things I got wrong about New York: that everyone was rich. I thought you needed to have money to have fun. But for dinner, Danielle and I went to Schiller's Liquor Bar—at the time, Keith McNally's newest gastropub. We split a hamburger and it was the most fun I'd had in ages. It was a Manhattan summer and the start of a great friendship. We were a perfect fashion couple. I wore pink ribbon belts. She wore boy shorts. We went to Fleet Week parties to gawk at Navy seamen let loose on New York, the mess of them dressed like the cast of *On the Town*. At night, I'd call Gary and tell him about the office and what had gone on there. I would tell him about the friends I was making and the stress of being an intern. I ate a lot of Chinese food from Baby Buddha, and I still crave it. As exciting as that time was, I think I was also a little lonely. But the work distracted me.

The *Vogue* office was as much our playground as it was our slave master. Long after the editors would go home at night, Danielle and I would stand in the fashion closet steaming dresses. In between chores, we'd play dress-up like deranged wannabe Cinderellas, taking Polaroids of ourselves wearing a Dior fur stole. I put on a Dior Russian fur hat and a Prada ombré shirt, and grasped a clutch. I like holding a purse in photos. A purse is the sign of a lady.

I was earning the trust of my superiors in the accessories closet, and soon I was taking black Lincoln Town Cars to Harry Winston to pick up jewelry valued in excess of $15 million. Me! Maybe it was my Canadian need to please others or the fact that I was older than the rest of the interns, but the editors seemed to trust me. And this kind of errand was not uncommon. I was regularly sent off to Lorraine Schwartz in the Diamond District to fetch jewels. Lorraine is famous for keeping Beyoncé and Jennifer Lopez in diamonds. Like any good Jewish mother, she is also famous for force-feeding those who enter her office with a good meal. This is how I ended up eating rotisserie chicken with Lorraine while looking at diamond rings. I was an intern carrying millions in jewels in my pockets without a security guard.

> "The *Vogue* office was as much our playground as it was our slave master."

And I was astonished that no security guard escorted me out. When I left, I simply kissed Lorraine good-bye and hopped back into the Town Car praying I wouldn't get mugged.

The summer passed by in a New York minute, and I was creating my own little fashion universe with Danielle and Annabet Duvall, then an assistant at *Jane,* whom I met at a birthday party at Max Fish. I wore a velvet blazer and a white shirt unbuttoned to my chest, my hair slicked down. It was too hot for that evening and the wrong outfit for a party on the Lower East Side, but it made quite an impression on people there. Yet while my internship was nearly over I had yet to go on a single shoot. I refused to give up. I'd come too far to quit. And I was in the elevator one day when I saw my chance. I don't know where the courage came from but there I was, riding the elevator with one of the *Vogue* editors, Jessica Diehl. I asked what she was doing for the weekend. She said she was stressing about a shoot she was styling for *Teen Vogue,* because she didn't have an assistant.

"If you need some help," I said, "let me know." I barely knew this woman, but she took me up on the offer and the next day I was at my first

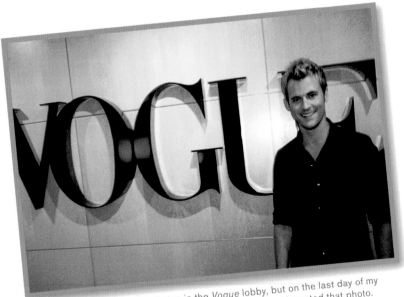

You're not supposed to take photos in the *Vogue* lobby, but on the last day of my internship, I broke down. If they were going to fire me, fine! I wanted that photo.

shoot, on set organizing shoes. She was even asking me questions. She'd say, "Is this cute?" Finally, I had a voice. I must have done something right, because a few days later, Grace Coddington's assistant, Michal Saad, asked me to assist on a Chanel shoot with the model Jessica Stam.

It was an out-of-body experience. Jessica Stam is a supermodel who matured in the Steven Meisel school of modeling. For *Vogue,* she was being shot outside the new Chanel store on Fifty-seventh Street for a page in a fall issue. We were seated inside an RV parked outside the store, and Jessica was having her makeup done. She had flaming red hair at the time, tucked underneath a wig—a blunt, brown bob not unlike Anna Wintour's own look. Jessica was Canadian, and while she was in hair and makeup, we laughed about Tim Hortons, a down-market Canadian coffee chain where Jessica was discovered at age fifteen. We laughed about the pig

Like a Virgin

OR HOW I MET MADONNA FOR THE FIRST TIME

When I was a kid, more than once I told my mom, "When I grow up, I'm going to meet Madonna." And at age twenty-three, I did. Let me set the scene: It was early 2003. I'd been living in L.A. for two years. Gary was writing for NBC's *Will & Grace* at the time, and Madge herself was scheduled to tape an appearance on the long-running sitcom. She hadn't agreed to take any photos with the crew or any of the guests. But Gary was determined to make that happen for me.

Our best shot was at this little meet-and-greet scheduled on the set after the taping of the episode. Gary knew the NBC on-set photographer and asked him earlier in the day if there was any way that he could try to orchestrate a photo with Madonna and me. And he did. Gary—so brave—approached Madonna. "My boyfriend is a huge fan of yours," he says. "Would you mind taking a photo with him?"

"If I take a photo with him, then I have to take a photo with everybody," Madonna said.

Meanwhile, I'm shaking. That was some serious kindergarten logic, but whatever. I thought, This isn't going to happen. Especially when Madonna's longtime PR rep, Liz Rosenberg, shuffled over. "What's going on here?" she said.

Suddenly the clouds parted, and Madonna—for reasons I'll never understand—had a change of heart.

"I'll take this one photo," she said.

I stepped forward. I told her I'm a huge fan. There wasn't much of a response, but I didn't mind. We turned toward the camera; I put my arm around her waist and Gary did the same. The photographer clicked the camera. And then he said, "Wait, I'm out of film."

I'm sure what happened next only lasted all of ten seconds.

(CONTINUED ON NEXT PAGE)

But in the moment, it felt like five minutes. My arm was still around Madonna's waist as the photographer threaded a new roll of film into the camera.

Finally, he snapped the photo. I had blond hair at the time. And I'd actually had a blow-out that morning. I'm so glad I have the photo. But I'm not happy that I look like Dana Carvey in *Wayne's World*.

farm in Ontario where she was born. It was cold outside on the street, and when we stepped out of the RV, Jessica wrapped her body around me for warmth. I felt the weight of a thousand eyes on me. Jessica Stam wasn't a household name yet, but people know when they are in the presence of extreme beauty. The boy inside me— the one who picked out clothing for his mother from the junk mail catalogs that came to the house—he could not believe that he was at a *Vogue* shoot with a supermodel on his arm, a supermodel who was dressed in a limited-edition, multicolored bouclé Chanel suit with a sheer ruffled blouse, an outfit designed specifically to mark the launch of this new store. (At the end of the shoot, the rep from Chanel gave her the suit as a gift. I thought, Holy fuck. I can't believe they just gave her a $15,000 suit.)

> "I remember feeling this burning sense of possibility. That there was more to my future than folding Hermès scarves in the windowless accessories closet."

I remember feeling this burning sense of possibility. That there was more to my future than folding Hermès scarves in the windowless accessories closet. This was only the beginning. This was only the first step. If I worked hard, I saw, if I was patient, good things would happen.

5

Fake it till you make it.
Yes, really.

IN FASHION CIRCLES, THE piece of advice thrown around most often is probably "Fake it till you make it." You know, pretend to know what you're doing and if you've got the goods, you'll figure it all out. This is also the only way to explain how, as a sophomore in college, I styled a newly famous Eva Longoria for the cover of *Life* magazine.

I had interned at *Vogue*. But in no way was I qualified—on paper or in the flesh—to style a cover shoot with a major star. However, through an unlikely turn of events, my childhood friend Tracy Doyle was now the photo director at the just-relaunched *Life* magazine. It was the fall of 2004, and *Life* was doing a yoga issue.

Desperate Housewives was an out-of-the-box hit for ABC, and while Eva Longoria was hot, she wasn't quite famous enough yet to demand her own stylist. Tracy vouched for me, and suddenly there I was, leaving class to pull looks from Juicy Couture and Lululemon and Bloomingdale's for a cover story with a legitimate magazine.

We'd be shooting at a house in Malibu Canyon, and before I left that morning, Gary said to me, "Remember, it's pronounced *Ee*-va, not *A*-va."

I repeated it back to him. "*Ee*-va," I said. "I know."

Of course the minute Ms. Longoria walked on set, I blurted out, "Hi, *A*-va, it's so nice to meet you."

She smiled at me, saying, "It's *Ee*-va." I winced and apologized. She said, "That's OK," and we walked back to look at the clothes together. We were shooting in the backyard, but because there were a couple of long-lens paparazzi hanging outside in the grass across the street, I had to set up the wardrobe racks inside the garage. Eva (not Ava!) perused the looks and more or less liked what I brought. I wasn't patting myself on the back. It was workout clothing, not couture gowns. Yet again, I was on the outside, scratching my way in. I was styling a major shoot, but it was jogging suits. There was definitely no Dior there.

> "I was on the outside, scratching my way in. I was styling a major shoot, but it was jogging suits. There was definitely no Dior there."

It wasn't all smooth sailing. Eva Longoria is a petite five foot two, and so the pants were all too long. At a *Vogue* shoot there would have been an on-set seamstress ready to work miracles. Here, we had Brad Goreski, college student, on his hands and knees trying to hem a starlet's velvet pants with duct tape.

Once we had the cover done and some inside looks shot, I tried to push the envelope, to bring a little glamour to this yoga story. For the final shot of the day, I dressed Eva in a metal, beaded gypsy skirt with a shirt tied and knotted at the waist to show off her taut stomach. She was lying down on a bunch of pillows. At the time it felt very cool. But I found a Polaroid of the shot recently (the image never ran in the magazine) and it looked like a catalog page from some Anthropologie knockoff. That fashion nightmare aside, the shoot was a success. We had a yoga specialist on set to assist with the poses, to make sure we didn't offend any actual yogis. I had to laugh six months later when I watched *The Comeback* on HBO. There was a similar scene with Valerie Cherish posing for the cover of *Be Yoga* magazine that hit a little too close to home.

The cover ran in January 2005 under the headline "Dogs do it, kids do it, even Desperate Housewives do it. Why we've become a Yoga Nation." Everyone at *Life* seemed pretty happy with it. Emboldened by my one bit of success, I sent that clip to every styling agency in L.A. the minute I got it, hoping to secure representation. (Celestine offered to put me on their list—of people to *assist* real stylists. Wah-wah.)

It was a ballsy move on my part. But I was a desperate housewife myself, desperate for a U.S. visa. The voices of Barbie and Marilyn and Claudia Schiffer were calling me. The *Vogue* internship only confirmed that I belonged in fashion. And yet, according to the U.S. government, I belonged in Canada.

> "It was a ballsy move on my part. But I was a desperate housewife myself, desperate for a U.S. visa."

I didn't have a green card. On my very first trip to Los Angeles straight from Greece, Gary and I had gone to see an immigration lawyer. This was not the kind of L.A. immigration lawyer that advertises in free Spanish-language newspapers. The office wasn't in Tijuana. We were in Beverly Hills, in a beautiful waiting room. Yet the law was pretty clear: As long as I was a student, I could stay in the country. After that, I'd need a full-time job and a company willing to sponsor my visa. This was no joke, and it was on my mind often and at odd times. In October of 2002, Gary and I went

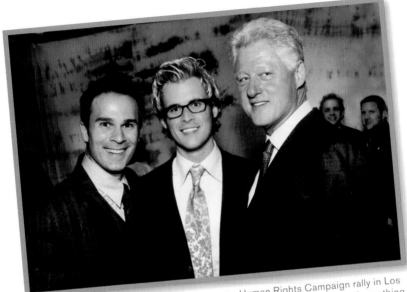

Gary and I met former president Bill Clinton at a Human Rights Campaign rally in Los Angeles. We're in matching Gucci. I have no idea what Bill is wearing. The funny thing is, he asked us to take this photo! You were supposed to pay extra to have your picture taken with Clinton. But we happened to be passing by just as the photographer passed by, and Clinton said, "Hey, guys! How about a picture!" True story.

to a Human Rights Campaign event honoring Bill Clinton. When we took a picture with him—both Gary and I in Gucci suits—I swear I thought about leaning over and asking Clinton to help me get a visa. I wasn't just fighting for employment. I was fighting for my life in Los Angeles. My life with Gary. Because, for the first time, I believed my life was worth fighting for. That *I* was worth fighting for.

Shortly after the *Life* magazine cover appeared on newsstands, my sister called: Our grandmother Ruby was sick with cancer and I should fly home immediately. Ruby—the woman who bought me Barbie dolls even though she knew my father would throw them out—had been sick for months. She knew her illness was serious, but she self-medicated with

Tylenol until the pain got so bad she had to see the doctor. The diagnosis was cancer, and she didn't have much time left.

We'd been in close touch over the years. My sponsor in AA had insisted I send regular letters to my grandmother as part of my amends, which I did. Sometimes these letters were substantial, other times they were just little note cards, reminders that I was out there and that I loved her and appreciated her. I'd call Ruby about my visa troubles, to tell her how stressed out I was. I was distraught, worried that the life Gary and I had created would be taken away from me. She told me, "We're a family of worriers. And that can't deter you. You can't let it destroy anything. Acknowledge that worrying is part of your personality. The world isn't out to get you." She was so happy for me and wanted me to snap out of it. She was always this way. When I was a kid, I'd say, "I can't wait for Christmas." She'd say, "Don't wish your life away." She was right. This was a precursor to AA. She was basically saying, "One day at a time."

> "For the first time, I believed my life was worth fighting for. That I was worth fighting for."

I'd seen her at Thanksgiving, and I'd been wearing a cashmere sweater she loved. Every time I passed by, she'd reach out to caress the soft wool. And so, for Christmas, my sister and I got her a cashmere blanket. She said she liked it, but, a spitfire to the end, she said she would have preferred a cashmere sweater. That was Ruby.

When my sister called to say that our grandmother's situation had worsened, I boarded a plane to Ontario, picking up a cashmere sweater for Ruby on the way—one last gift so she knew what she meant to me. So she knew I owed her everything. When she opened the box and held up the sweater, she said it was the nicest thing she'd ever owned in her life. She wanted to be buried in it, she said, and when she passed away a few days later, we honored her request. Back at the house, I found a stack of the letters I'd sent her over the years, tucked away next to her favorite chair.

One of her friends told me that Ruby would read these notes again and again. She called them her "love letters."

Grandma Ruby's passing focused me. I was in the hospital with her when she died. I remember looking around the room and feeling grateful that I was there. Grateful that I was physically allowed to be in the room when she passed. If I'd still been using drugs, I would have missed this entirely. And even if I'd made it to the hospital, in the state I was in when I was using, no one would have let me near my grandmother. But now I felt strong. I felt like a man. I wanted to continue on this path, to be a better person. For me. For Gary. But also for Ruby.

> "I felt like a man. I wanted to continue on this path, to be a better person. For me. For Gary. But also for Ruby."

These words went through my head: Look around you. Take notes. Prepare yourself for what is next. Because what is next is your life. It is waiting for you.

I transferred to USC in 2006 and majored in art history. When I was at *Vogue,* I was often photocopying historical references from art books. The editors would flag old images as inspiration shots. Camilla Nickerson and Grace Coddington would have art books open all the time. If I'm going to be a stylist, I thought, I should know painters and photographers and color composition and how it all fits together. And I worked hard. I was diligent in my studies, but more than that, I was focused on gaining actual real-world experience. Herein, a fast-forward flip book through my grunt work.

I was back in New York the summer after my *Vogue* internship, interning this time at *W* magazine. I was obsessed with the fashion and style editor Alex White, who consistently pushed the boundaries of what an American fashion magazine could be with shoots that were as

Required Reading

SEVEN MUST-HAVE FASHION COFFEE TABLE BOOKS

1. *Blood Sweat and Tears,* Bruce Weber (1999)
This iconic photographer captures the kind of teenage years I wish
I'd lived: beautiful, topless girls in the Hamptons with the hottest
surfer guys around.

**2. *The Costume History,* Auguste Racinet (1876; reissued by
Taschen paperback in 2009)**
Fashion plates and historical references. Do your homework!
Alexander McQueen was obsessed with the Victorian era and
the Scottish Highlands. John Galliano was obsessed with corset
construction. Those original references—for silhouettes, for
shapes—are all here.

3. *Tom Ford,* Tom Ford (2008)
From Tom Ford's years at YSL to Gucci to his own eponymous
label, it's all here. Think modern sexuality. Think smoldering. Think
of the Gucci G shaved into a girl's pubic hair.

**4. *Grace: Thirty Years of Fashion at Vogue,* Grace
Coddington (2002)**
No explanation necessary.

5. *Rock and Royalty,* Gianni Versace (1997)
Gianni Versace's couture, featuring Linda, Christy, Naomi, and a
continuation of the excess of the eighties into the next decade.
Genius.

**6. *Minimalism and Fashion: Reduction in the Postmodern
Era*, Elyssa Dimant (2010)**
A retrospective of minimalism—huge in the nineties, and back
again now.

(CONTINUED ON NEXT PAGE)

7. *Helmut Newton: Polaroids*, Helmut Newton (2011)
Known for his disturbing and overt sexuality, Helmut Newton
created some of the most lasting images of women. His shots of
Nadja Auermann haunt me. When I was in high school, I remember
seeing Newton's shots of Nadja in *Vogue*. Nadja is known for her
legs. And so he shot her in leg braces and on crutches, walking
down the stairs in a pencil skirt. Arresting.

high-fashion as European editorials but still palatable on U.S. shores. I
especially loved one shoot where she dressed men in women's clothing.
It was shocking to see real men in heels on the cover of an American
magazine. There was an air of mystery about it, like we'd been transported
to some secret society somewhere. There's more: I was obsessed with a
Karen Elson shoot Alex styled—an iconic series taken on soaking-wet
Manhattan streets. She has a specific eye, telling stories with the collections
but always making them her own. She is like Grace Coddington in that
respect. I wanted to know how that brain works.

Unfortunately, the summer that I interned at *W,* Alex White was
out on maternity leave, and my sole interaction with her consisted of one
afternoon when I dropped a package off at her front door. Typical! Though
I should say, even that one moment was memorable, because when she
opened the door, she was wearing a monogrammed denim Louis Vuitton
dress—one of *the* key pieces of the season.

Still, the job was a learning experience. For *W,* we shot a post–*Donnie
Darko,* pre–*Brokeback Mountain* Jake Gyllenhaal. I didn't know who he
was. But my girlfriends were freaking out, begging me for Polaroids from
the shoot. What I remember more than the styling that day is Jake and
Kirsten Dunst. The two were dating at the time, and after the shoot, they
sat together at Milk Studios sipping champagne. It all felt too glamorous.

Art School Confidential

TEN ARTISTS YOU SHOULD KNOW

1. Kara Walker

Her oversize silhouettes are a sometimes shocking commentary on the antebellum South. Stop, look, and contemplate. These images are meant to start a dialogue about racial relationships.

2. Nikki S. Lee

This Korean-American photographer is known for a series called *Projects,* where she immerses herself in different societies, capturing cultures with a point-and-click camera and a time/date stamp. It's deceptively simple. She's a voyeur—whether she's hanging out in a trailer park or with senior citizens—and by extension, so are we. I dream of owning a Nikki S. Lee print.

3. François Boucher

A French painter in the eighteenth century, Boucher did a series of detailed portraits of Madame de Pompadour—Louis XV's chief mistress from 1745 to her death in 1764. She was one of my obsessions in school. To me, Madame de Pompadour is all about decadence. She was a tastemaker and Boucher captures that spirit wonderfully.

4. Ernst Kirchner

A great example of German Expressionism, Kirchner's *Street, Dresden* is one of my favorite paintings, and I stop in to see it every time I'm at the MoMA. The palette is beautiful, as is the scale.

5. Constantin Brancusi

A Romanian-born sculptor. His *Bird in Flight* is the definition of modernity.

(CONTINUED ON NEXT PAGE)

6. Robert Mapplethorpe
One of the most important photographers dealing with male sexuality and homosexuality—period.

7. Mark Rothko
Sitting in a room surrounded by Rothko paintings gives me a particular sensation—it's like the room is throbbing. His humming energy comes through the paintings and penetrates your body.

8. Florian Maier-Aichen
The Blum & Poe Gallery in L.A. handles this young artist's work—these beautiful, moody large-scale landscape photographs that take up almost an entire wall. I don't know if I have a wall large enough in my house to accommodate one, but that's the dream!

9. Michelangelo
I know, not a surprise. But I've seen *David* on three separate trips to Florence, and he never ceases to amaze.

10. Gian Lorenzo Bernini
An Italian artist from the seventeenth century, Bernini is perhaps best known for his sculpture *Apollo and Daphne,* which depicts a scene from Ovid's *Metamorphoses* in which a woman becomes a tree. This must be seen up close to truly appreciate the intricate and delicate detail, and also the emotion. The leaves and twigs are growing out of Daphne's hands—and it's this massive rush of energy.

In many ways, Alex's assistant, Marina Burini, was running the show and everyone lived in fear of her. She was very French in appearance, wearing mostly black dresses that fell below the knee and sensible sandals. She was the assistant to the queen bee and her voice mattered. But Marina was also under a lot of pressure, trying to pull all of these complicated fashion shoots together without the boss. At the time, I didn't really understand the stress she was under. It wasn't until years later, when I was working for Rachel Zoe, that I really understood the logistics she was up against. Yet Marina rarely, if ever, let anyone see her sweat.

I was afraid of Marina, too, I should say. Afraid every time she crossed my path in the office. But I was nobody's bitch that summer. There was less of an established hierarchy at *W* than at *Vogue,* and I was hands-on at photo shoots. I wasn't just observing how the parts moved. I was actually doing the job. I was getting messy, sometimes quite literally. I was at a shoot one afternoon steaming a satin dress. I had no idea what I was doing, mind you, and water was splashing everywhere, threatening to ruin this very expensive, handmade dress. Marina saw what was happening and stopped what she was doing. I thought I was going to get yelled at, but

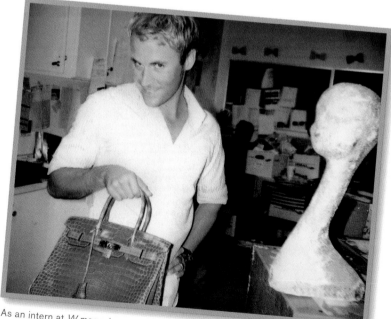

As an intern at *W* magazine, I couldn't help but pose with this $50,000 magenta Birkin bag. There was a massive waiting list for the Birkin back then—there still is—and I had to hold it.

instead she took the time to show me the proper way to steam a dress. "Pull the fabric tight," she said, instructing me, "and steam from the inside, not the outside." She also told me that if you put a sock over the head of the steamer, it'll help stem the sputtering water.

It's not just practical skills I took from Marina. I learned the importance of photo shoot etiquette. One day, I was assisting at a shoot for Swarovski that Marina was styling. Guinevere van Seenus was the model—which made me laugh, because I knew Guinevere. Not from New York fashion parties, not from the fashion world at all, but because she sat in front of me in French class at Santa Monica College. We greeted each other like old friends, and during lunch, we caught up. Craig McDean, a world-class photographer, was shooting that day's Swarovski story, and he joined us for lunch. The three of us were talking about who knows what when Marina appeared out of nowhere, leaned in, and whispered in my ear, "Can I talk to you for a second?" Uh-oh.

> "I was caught off guard by her question. This dragon lady, this woman I'd been terrified of, had that much faith in me?"

I excused myself from the table, never to return. Marina explained that when a photographer sits down with his subject, the assistants are meant to disappear. The photographer needs that time to establish a rapport with the talent. Everyone else—even if you are old college friends—is simply in the way. Lesson learned.

Marina was nearing the end of her stint with Alex White—there is a natural time for every assistant to move on—and she was looking for a replacement. Even though I was only a junior in college, Marina asked if I might be interested in the job. She had been interviewing people and giving people trial runs, but no one had really worked out. But she saw something in me, she said. She asked if I would stay on, shadow her when Alex returned, and see if it was a good fit.

I was caught off guard by her question. This dragon lady, this woman

Take Care (of Your Clothing)

HOW TO MAKE WHAT'S IN YOUR CLOSET LAST

1. Don't over-dry-clean things. I wear my suits a few times before I send them to the dry cleaners. Instead of protecting your clothes, the chemicals in dry cleaning can actually start wearing the fabric down. Unless you have a stain or unwanted scent, I suggest wearing it a few times.
2. Moths: Invest in cedar disks for the tops of your hangers to keep the moths away.
3. If you're going to spend $600 on a pair of shoes—and I have a weakness for expensive shoes—invest in shoe trees to preserve them. I love patent leather, which can tend to get wrinkly, but a shoe tree will help the shoe keep its shape and prevent creases in the leather.
4. Use a furniture spray like Endust to shine your patent leather.
5. Give your clothes room to breathe. Do not keep them all jammed together. It's hard to find things and not good for the longevity of your clothes. If this is happening, it's time to consider editing your closet.
6. Keep very fragile or expensive items of clothing in garment bags and/or plastic. This is a no-brainer.

I'd been terrified of, had that much faith in me? Over the summer, she'd welcomed me into the fold, and this introduction meant more to me than she could ever have known. I discussed the potential opportunity with Gary and we even talked to an immigration lawyer, who advised me to stay in school instead and get my degree. It was not an easy decision. This was the first time in my life that I felt almost on the inside. But I took the lawyer's advice and went back to school, as hard as that was.

I worried: What if I give up this job at *W,* and an opportunity like it never comes again? I convinced myself this fear was irrational; I had

You Better *Work*

HOW TO GET A SUMMER INTERNSHIP IN FASHION

1. Identify the job.

As Fraulein Maria says in *The Sound of Music,* let's start at the very beginning. Where do you want to work? Dream big. Don't worry about who you know or don't know. Just make the list. And know what you're going after.

2. Be resourceful.

When I started looking for internships, I barely had my own e-mail address. But it's a whole new world now. Be resourceful. If you want to work at a fashion magazine, open up the book and find the masthead. E-mail someone whose work you admire. Or better yet, e-mail their assistant. Go on Facebook. Go on Twitter. Also: Don't forget the original, classic route. Pick up the phone and call the human resources department. Condé Nast has a formal internship program. So does Hearst. Find the application online, and find it early.

3. Dress up.

You'll need a stroke of luck to land a job. I get that. But you need to be prepared when that luck strikes. And that means being presentable when you walk through the door. I tend to think it's better to overdress for an interview. In fashion especially, no one wants to hire a slob. Be well dressed—whatever that means to you. When I interviewed with Anna Wintour at *Vogue,* I wore a wool Gucci suit even though it was the dead of summer. I kept my shit together. Wear something that shows you can dress yourself.

4. Do your homework.

Internships are so competitive these days, you need to show that you really want it. The best way to do that is to study up on the company. Know the magazine. Know the photographers who shoot for the magazine. Know the writers and editors by name, so you can reference their work. Internships lay the foundation for your future success. This homework is an investment. Also, know what to expect from the job. Know that you're not going to be hanging out with the boss, sipping cocktails on a summer afternoon in the Hamptons. Understand that you'll be doing grunt work, and be excited to learn from that work.

5. Send a handwritten thank-you note.
Preferably on personalized stationery, which everyone should have. If not, go to a stationery store and buy a set of nice cards. Crane makes beautiful ones for $10. Spend a little extra. They'll notice the paper stock. And your stock will rise.

to. I needed to believe the work would come. This would not be my only chance at bat. It helped that Tracy Doyle, who hired me for the *Life* magazine shoot, sent another job my way. I styled a shoot for *Time Out New York* celebrating the top ten bars in the five boroughs. A male and female model posed as a couple in each bar, and I dressed them for a series of first dates. It was a more complicated shoot than it sounds. Each image was set in a different period. For a 1970s mai tai photograph, I dressed the female model in a Diane von Furstenberg wrap dress. For the eighties, it was a vintage Lacroix moment. For the 1990s, it was Gaultier. I pulled everything myself from (among other places) a vintage supplier in SoHo, What Goes Around Comes Around. I had no assistant, no budget. It was just me running around the city with garbage bags full of clothes. Still, it was a credit. It was a notch on my studded Gucci belt.

There were more milestones, more victories—personally and professionally. There was always farther to go. My path was wide open. I stayed in Los Angeles the next summer, interning with Cristina Ehrlich and Estee Stanley, two well-known celebrity stylists who worked with Penélope Cruz and Reese Witherspoon, among others. I was thrown into the deep end. Their assistant was eight months pregnant and she trained me for a week before disappearing. I helped Cristina and Estee with their fashion line, Miss Davenport. I did a fitting at Jessica Biel's house. Biel was promoting *The Illusionist,* a prestige film she made with Edward Norton. She did a British accent in the film, and the well-reviewed piece would help establish Biel as much more than the girl from *7th Heaven* with the perfect body. Though she was that, too, which I found out on our first meeting. I'd come to her house for the fitting. I knocked on the door, but there was no answer. I knocked

> "She was soaking wet, wearing nothing but a string bikini. I realize this is a male fantasy. But not *this* male's fantasy."

again and heard her yell from the back of the house, "I'm coming." And then Jessica Biel, Hollywood bombshell, opened the front door to her house coming fresh from the pool. She was soaking wet, wearing nothing but a string bikini. I realize this is a male fantasy. But not *this* male's fantasy.

"Where can I set up?" I said, itching to drop the garment bags that were weighing down my hands.

I was five years sober when I called Nick. It was time to make amends. I flew to Toronto and we met on Yonge Street at Le Marche, a restaurant where we used to go on weekends. It was hard to face him. When I looked back on the relationship, I realized how much I'd pointed my finger and blamed him for my falling off the wagon, for us not working out. That was the hardest part for me to deal with. To see the damage I'd done from his perspective. He'd welcomed me into his home and I'd bulldozed through like a storm, running through the house tearing stuff up. Our relationship got bad because I made it bad. There were times when he acted out, yes. But it was a manifestation of the world I'd created. Sitting there at the café five years later, he looked older but still handsome. What I'll always remember is the look of relief that came across his face. That I acknowledged my part. But also that I was not just on my feet but happy. The relief came from me, as well. I'd been struggling for years with how I'd apologize. This was keeping me back from moving forward. The five-year mark was a perfect time to let that go. And to allow Nick to let go.

I graduated from USC in 2008 with a degree in art history. I was twenty-five years old. And I needed an entry-level job. I had an idea of what this job would be: I wanted to work for Rachel Zoe. The only problem was, we hadn't met yet.

I had been trying to track down Rachel Zoe for months. If you aspire to be a celebrity stylist in Los Angeles, then you dream of training under Rachel. She was the first stylist to be in French *Vogue*—in her own feature, not styling someone else. She dressed Keira Knightley for the 2006 Academy Awards in a burgundy Vera Wang gown (which, rumor has it, Rachel had a hand in designing herself). Either way, the dress was perfection. The truth is, no one knew what a stylist *was* until Rachel came along. She made it a legitimate career. If I was going to dedicate myself to someone for three years,

> "I had an idea of what this job would be: I wanted to work for Rachel Zoe. The only problem was, we hadn't met yet."

about the length of time for a job like that—and I didn't want to be some tragic thirty-eight-year-old stylist assistant—I wanted to do it with Rachel.

But I needed a personal introduction. I couldn't find anyone who knew her, and believe me, I was relentless in my pursuit. Neither of her assistants was on Facebook. Twitter didn't exist yet. I dropped her name every chance I got, hoping that by putting it out into the universe, the universe would send back a sign. Which is sort of what happened. In the end, it was the spirit of Coco Chanel that would bring us together.

I was at the Kasdan mansion on November 7, 2006, at a dinner in Beverly Hills celebrating the launch of Chanel's fine jewelry collection. It was a sensible party for 250 people. So sensible, in fact, that there was a miniature train set winding through the backyard. There were several Picassos in the house as well, and a burly security guard standing watch. How did I come to be at this dinner? I certainly wasn't invited on my own, at least not by the House of Chanel. Yes, I'd styled Eva Longoria for the yoga issue of *Life* magazine, but that wasn't opening these guilded doors. What happened was a lot less glamorous: Gary's agent's wife needed a date and for Chanel, I would make myself available. My date's name was Candie. And so I wore Gary's chocolate-brown Dolce & Gabbana three-piece suit.

I'd like to pause to say how strange the universe is: Candie could have taken anyone to this party. This was a major fashion event in Beverly Hills, and Candie was über-stylish. She was a big wearer of head-to-toe Chanel. She'd wear thigh-high Chanel boots with perfect hair and crazy jewelry. She was super-high-fashion. When Gary and I first got together, before I ever had my own career going, I always looked forward to

> "Gary's agent's wife needed a date and for Chanel, I would make myself available."

seeing Candie at parties, especially at her house. While the other wives were downstairs, Candie and I would be in her closet looking through the Chanel. She was one of the few people I knew in L.A. who was really into fashion. And the fact that she invited me to this party touched me. She could have taken one of her husband's famous clients. She could have taken anyone, really. But she chose to take me—a client's boyfriend who was in school at USC but who she knew would truly appreciate it. And I did.

At the dinner, Candie introduced me to Elizabeth Stewart, a stylist for the *New York Times Magazine*. I told her that I'd just finished an internship with Cristina and Estee (that's how they're known in the industry) and that I had a premonition that I was going to work for Rachel Zoe. If only I could meet her.

"I know Rachel Zoe!" Elizabeth said. "She's coming tonight. I'll introduce you."

"Really?" I said.

"Of course!"

Moments later, as if on cue, Rachel walked in with Nicole Richie. Rachel was dressed in a black, long-sleeved chiffon maxi dress. But the first thing I noticed was her eyes and how big they were. She was straying from her tan boho thing, and this new look was working for her. She looks like Barbie, I thought. Like a real Barbie. I was in awe.

Elizabeth grabbed me. I tried to be demure. "No, no, no," I said, chickening out.

"It's a great opportunity," she said. "Tell her you want to be her assistant."

> "She looks like Barbie, I thought. Like a real Barbie. I was in awe."

And so I did. I told Rachel that I was finishing school and if she ever needed help I'd love to work for her. She told me to get her assistant's e-mail address from Elizabeth and to keep in touch. Keep in touch? Well, I took those three little words as an invitation to politely stalk her.

Meanwhile, Nicole Richie was smiling courteously while I networked. Her hair was brown and pulled up in a loose bun with bangs in front of her face. She said something about my being cute. (Thanks!) And then—because this night couldn't get any weirder—a photographer from WireImage materialized out of thin air and captured the whole thing on film. Or digital, at least. I don't know what he was shooting with.

The next morning, I called Tracy at her office in New York.

"Do you have a WireImage account?" I asked.

"Yes."

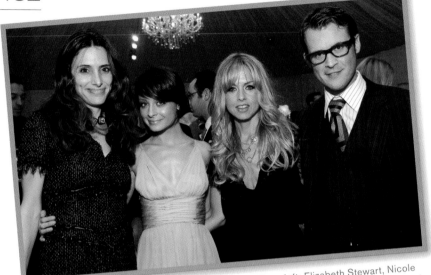

Photographic evidence of the night I met Rachel Zoe. From left: Elizabeth Stewart, Nicole Richie, Rachel Zoe, and one very surprised Brad Goreski. I don't know who the photographer thought I was (because I wasn't anybody). But I'm certainly glad to have this photo.

"You have to buy the photo of me and Rachel Zoe."

I proceeded to e-mail every single person I knew to relate this story; it was such an extreme high. Of course all extreme highs are followed by extreme lows. As directed, I e-mailed Rachel's assistant, who quickly replied to say that no positions were available at the House of Zoe but she'd "keep my résumé on file." Keep my résumé on file? That didn't sound very promising.

Not to be deterred, I sent this woman an e-mail every three weeks, asking if anything had changed. When I had a break from school, I sent an e-mail. "If you ever need an extra set of hands," I wrote, "let me know and I'll be there!" I thought I'd continue to do this until I was told not to or until Rachel hired someone else. Whichever came first. In the meantime, I told anyone I knew in fashion to mention my name to Rachel, so that I would be constantly on her brain. And through yet another strange cosmic coincidence, Tracy left *Life* magazine to work as photographer Steven Klein's producer. She met Rachel on a Brad Pitt shoot in Prague and told her that she had to hire me. That her friend was desperate to work for her.

And still . . . nothing. Did I mention I really needed a job? That was when I heard of an opening at *Vogue*'s West Coast office, as the Los Angeles sittings assistant. I applied and Condé Nast flew me to New York for an interview with Her Majesty Anna Wintour. I wore a navy blue striped Gucci suit with a blue-and-white-striped collared banker shirt and cherry-colored Gucci slip-ons. I wore this suit because it fit well, but more important because it looked expensive. When I came face-to-face with Anna for the first time, it was like seeing the Sasquatch. (It exists!) She was wearing a beige skirt and a twinset and a pair of Manolo mules— sunglasses off for the interview. I was told that she'd be in a good mood because her friend Roger Federer had won some tennis match the night before, and the intel proved to be true. She smiled. She probed. She asked me about the differences between West Coast and East Coast fashion. I answered with something about how the two influence each other, which she seemed to like. I made her laugh, which felt like the biggest victory. We shook hands (physical contact!). Everything was shaking, actually. I was exhilarated yet terrified. I had dreamed of this moment my whole life, and I was just pleased that I didn't mess it up. I flew back to Los Angeles feeling content, feeling a sense of promise.

> "When I came face-to-face with Anna for the first time, it was like seeing the Sasquatch. (It exists!)"

While I was waiting to hear from Condé Nast, an e-mail arrived from Rachel asking me to come in for an interview—out of the blue. It was July of 2008 and she was thinking of hiring a third assistant. I'd made an impression on her, she said, and she wanted to talk. Unfortunately, the position would only be part-time but I scheduled the interview anyway. I wore a blue, vintage pin-striped vest and a white shirt, and a burgundy patterned Gucci tie and jeans—despite the fact that it was boiling out. I realized the minute I walked in that I was overdressed. Rachel was in wide-leg faded 7 For All Mankind jeans and an off-the-shoulder Stella McCartney T-shirt and so much jewelry I wasn't entirely sure how her neck was supporting it all. Taylor Jacobson—the blonde who would later become my nemesis on national television—was dressed in a sweat suit, with sunglasses and a black T-shirt.

I was walking into a minefield. We sat down for the interview and Taylor was on the phone with Lindsay Lohan's assistant, yelling about some Chloé dress they couldn't find. Rachel's assistant Leah did most of the talking. I can't remember what we talked about. I just remember that Taylor was on her BlackBerry the entire time. She wasn't engaged at all. She was only there because Rachel wanted her in the room. But we barely made eye contact. Of course I was thinking to myself, I've been waiting a year for this interview and you can't take your sunglasses off? You can't stop yelling about some dress Lindsay Lohan can't find? This is my moment and you're talking over it!

But Taylor surprised me, and we had a real person-to-person moment as I was walking out. Before I could leave, she stopped me to say, "I'll be seeing you soon, I'm sure."

"What does that mean?" I asked.

"Rachel really liked you," Taylor said. "I can tell."

While she was right, it was too little too late. Rachel called to offer me a part-time position and it was bittersweet. Yes, it would have been a foot in the door. But there was no guarantee of anything permanent, and I panicked: Maybe it's just not meant to be. Maybe I'm not meant to work for Rachel. In the same breath, Condé Nast called to offer me the full-time position at *Vogue*'s West Coast office, and I accepted the job, starting immediately. I harbored the hope that if I proved myself at *Vogue,* someone at the magazine might sponsor my visa.

I was walking away from Rachel. Little did I know that I'd be walking right back soon enough.

6

Open your eyes.

TO BE AN ASSISTANT at *Vogue* is to be perched on the lowest rung of a very tall, very stylish totem pole. And as the West Coast assistant, I was doing a lot of administrative work. I was filing expense reports and organizing receipts and sending flowers to everyone in the fashion world. We had a regular, *Vogue*-approved florist and I talked to him more than I talked to Gary. This guy recently Facebooked me. "You used to call me all the time!" he said. Because I did.

I was not above grunt work. I just wished I was good at it. Our phone system wasn't all that complicated, but I don't think I ever correctly put a call through to Lisa Love, our West Coast editor. It was a joke. One day I picked up the phone and the voice on the other end said, "It's Anna." All I could think was, Don't get this wrong. *Don't hang up on Anna Wintour!*

Some people are lucky enough to have that double skill set—to be able to organize a life and do Excel spreadsheets and handle receipts. But that wasn't me. I was at *Vogue*, which was a dream come true. But once again I was still not quite at the party. Lisa Love and Lawren Howell were a dream to work for. But I wanted to be touching the clothes. And most of that happens in New York.

As part of my job, I was also the liaison to the magazine's New York office, and I helped in any way I could. Some *Vogue* staffers think that traveling to Los Angeles is like going to Japan. They don't know how to navigate this crazy place with palm trees and traffic, and it was my job to facilitate their visits. I organized armored trucks for jewelry. I sat on Lisa Love's floor counting out three hundred pieces of jewelry. Costume jewelry, meanwhile, would arrive with a stone missing. A Marni necklace would show up with a broken clasp. Cataloging the incoming jewelry was nerve-racking work, because anything that was missing was my fault. I'd call the New York office and explain that a certain piece arrived damaged. Invariably they'd say, "Well, it didn't leave the New York office that way. Did something happen when you opened the package?"

I flew to New York for Fashion Week, and Danielle—my best friend from the summer I spent interning at *Vogue,* the one who went with me to all of those Fleet Week parties—was now a fashion assistant at *T,* the *New York Times*'s fashion magazine. While we worked at two of the most respected publications in the industry, no one in the industry knew our names. We begged for fashion show tickets and were often turned away. When we did manage to get tickets by some Harry Potter fashion magic, we were standing in the back craning our necks.

There is one show we don't have to beg our way into: Our friend Annabet Duvall launched her own line, Doucette Duvall, and she was having a presentation in the Meatpacking District. It was major. A *Vogue*

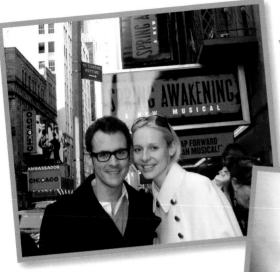

Whenever I'd come to New York, I'd see at least one Broadway show. I saw *Spring Awakening* five times. I was obsessed with Lea Michele long before *Glee*. To me, this was the new *Rent*. This was the musical the next generation would be talking about to define their late teens and early twenties.

This is the first night I wore a bow tie. I was in New York, and Annabet Duvall and I went to Arena. It was so hot that night, but I refused to take off my black cashmere Marc Jacobs sweater, because I thought I'd look like a waiter. But it was a big hit.

threesome—Sally Singer, Virginia Smith, and Lauren Santo Domingo—was there. The clothing was flirty, with a touch of country girl. But the presentation had a masculine bent, with vignettes set at a polo club and one at a cigar bar. The models had strong brows and wore bright colors—blues and yellows and big greens dominated. Playing off the color pops in the show, there were goodie bags filled with M&M's for everyone. I hadn't told Annabet I was coming to town, and it was amazing to surprise her. After the presentation, Danielle and I walked south and hit West Broadway arm in arm. The weather was gorgeous, a perfect Manhattan fall day, all brisk air and bright sunshine. We were standing on a street corner in SoHo laughing about this world we lived in, about how far we'd come from the *Vogue* internships three years ago and yet how far we had to go. We tore into the bag of candy and M&M's fell all over the street.

> " This moment would forever define us: It was the realization of just how far we had to climb. Though we didn't know this yet, there would come a day when we wouldn't have to beg to get a ticket to a fashion show. "

We ate the few pieces of candy we managed to save and we laughed, because we felt like losers. This moment would forever define us: It was the realization of just how far we had to climb. Though we didn't know this yet, there would come a day when we wouldn't have to beg to get a ticket to a fashion show. Yet every time we walked into the tents together, for years to come, Danielle and I would always ask each other, "Do you have your M&M's?"

While in New York, I assisted *Vogue*'s Lawren Howell on a portfolio of CFDA Award finalists. She could have used a New York assistant, but she used me. We shot Liya Kebede and Peter Som at a haunting mansion on Long Island that was frozen in time. There was no heat and we were shivering but the project was like a jolt in the arm. I was filled with a sense of purpose. This little taste of the fashion world was enough to make me feel like I was a part of something larger. That action was enough to keep me going.

I was back in Los Angeles when a saving grace arrived—in the form of Grace Coddington.

It was November 2007, and Grace, the legendary creative director of American *Vogue*, was flying out from New York for a three-day fashion shoot at Frank Sinatra's onetime home in the San Fernando Valley, where he often held court with the Rat Pack. Sinatra moved into the home in 1945 and recorded a song about the Valley. The lyrics: *"'cause I've decided where yours truly should be, and it's the San Fernando Valley for me."* And that day it was for me as well. Mario Testino was shooting. The model Karen Elson, then married to Jack White of the White Stripes, was the star. In short, it was major.

If I was nervous that day, it had everything to do with Grace Coddington. Not because of her reputation as a demanding perfectionist, but because I was obsessed with her. Grace grew up in a tiny town in Wales, so remote she'd have to send away for copies of *Vogue;* the magazines would arrive three months after their on-sale date. At age seventeen, she won a modeling contest and suddenly found herself in the pages of the very magazine she'd worshipped all those years. She was stunning—a vision of pale, frizzy red hair. Helmut Newton shot Grace more than once. Devastatingly, at age twenty-six, Grace was in a car accident in which she lost an eyelid, thus cutting her modeling career short. She was not done with fashion, though. Hardly. Grace worked for British *Vogue* for nineteen years and eventually made her way to American *Vogue,* where she and Anna Wintour started work within days of each other. She is Anna's right-hand woman, the Gayle to Anna's Oprah, as anyone who saw the documentary *The September Issue* knows. Where Anna is a vision of extreme control, Grace is as fiery as her red hair, a wild and woolly mane that is her signature and her armor all at once. I remember buying her book, *Grace: Thirty Years of Fashion at Vogue,* just before my internship and flipping through the pages, wondering how I could get on set with one of the biggest legends in the fashion world.

I didn't expect that I'd have much interaction with Grace on this shoot, of course. My job that day was to help Grace's assistant, Sonya, with whatever she needed. Still, I got to watch. We showed up at the Sinatra estate and the first thing I noticed wasn't the period-perfect kitchen or the beautiful gardens, but rather Grace's concise fashion edit. This is a woman who knows what she likes. There were only four racks of clothing. The theme for the shoot was 1950s glamour, which would have been obvious to anyone who saw her edit. There was Dior (tight fitted tops and full-skirted silhouettes) and Marc Jacobs (pointy-toed pumps with ostrich bows) and pairs of cat-eye glasses. There were floral rubber bathing caps by Marni and skinny belts, cardigans, and gloves. There was no on-the-fly tinkering here, no boiling down of the looks on set to a central message. That work had already been painstakingly done back in New York.

Mario Testino arrived on set and breezed through like a cloud of effervescent smoke. He was the definition of charming. Not to mention seriously funny. And he interacted with everyone, his quick laugh making even the catering hands feel essential and—more important—feel beautiful. Having met him, it's clear how he gets the likes of Angelina Jolie to disrobe for his lens.

I had my marching orders for this three-day shoot: I was to be seen and not heard. And for the bulk of the time, that was how it went. Until Sonya needed me on set. There I was holding a tray of sunglasses in my arms, like a soldier at the ready. Watching Grace on set is like taking a master class in the importance of fine details. Grace placed Karen Elson in an open bedroom doorway, the two French doors ajar. Karen was dressed in a strapless metallic blue Nina Ricci dress, with Marc Jacobs silk gloves. It was one of my favorite looks from that season's Nina Ricci collection. Grace placed Karen's hands against the door. Gorgeous light came into the room directly over Karen's shoulder, bathing her in a lush glow.

"*Divino*," Mario said.

But Grace was still fiddling. Mario brought a childlike energy with him, but Grace was the taskmaster. They worked in tandem, like a well-oiled glamour machine. Grace was dressed in workmanlike Prada, black slacks and a white top, and she was a mercenary of precision. She was posing Karen like the most beautiful paper doll, instructing her how to hold her body. The direction was hyper-specific: Move your hand down half an inch and turn your body a quarter of an inch. These were not casual whims. Grace could see the frame, she could see how the photograph would be laid out in the pages of *Vogue*. Her eye is so trained, she can see the shot before it's taken. Standing at the back of the room, I thought, I have never seen Karen Elson look so beautiful as she does today in this light. I want to see what Grace sees. I want to know what she knows.

It was a rare moment of calm on the set. Later, Grace was running around saying there were too many people at the shoot. There were assistants hanging out by the catering all day and she went ballistic. One of the production assistants was some L.A. surfer dude with his hair pulled back into a blond ponytail and wearing Dickies pants. Grace kept asking people what he did. "He's always eating," she said. "Why is he always eating? What is he doing here?"

Grace is old-school. She comes from a time where you'd go to the Australian outback with a crew of five, and you'd be carrying the clothes yourself and everyone would be pulling double duty, collaborating together trying to make beautiful photos. Now there are seventy-five people on set and you don't know who is doing what. Grace is also one of the few major stylists who is still so hands-on. She jokes that she's one of the last who still touches the model herself. Now here was this Spicoli-type dude raiding the craft services table.

I was in fear of being evicted from the set. More than that, I wanted Grace to like me. This was a special opportunity. And I was so desperately trying to look busy, desperately trying to earn my keep. That's one thing I learned as an intern: Always look busy. There's always something that needs straightening. Something always needs fixing.

And so I started steaming skirts, straightening accessories, organizing the bags—anything to stay in the frame myself. There was a custom Gucci dress Grace was expecting that day, a dress that was stuck at the airport in customs. (I know the feeling.) And so I called Worldnet, the courier service of choice for fashion, every fifteen minutes to see when we could expect that dress to show up. The whole day was about that dress. "Where is the Gucci?" Grace kept asking.

When the dress finally materialized, the moment was decidedly anticlimactic. Grace took one look at the dress hanging on the rack, said, "This isn't going to work," and walked away. Oh, well.

At this point, I was fairly certain Grace and I would not speak. Which was fine. It was enough that I saw her and Mario Testino collaborate. That was enough of a lesson to make this entire job at *Vogue* worthwhile. These were the moments I lived for. And it certainly beat sending flowers.

> "It takes a village to raise a fashion story."

I was continuing to fiddle on set, continuing to earn my keep, when I noticed a cream, halter-neck Donna Karan dress with a cinched waist and a full skirt, very Marilyn Monroe in *The Seven Year Itch,* hanging on a rack. I remembered the dress from the look book. It was all big silk chiffon, and it had been terribly flattened out in transport. Now the dress looked sad. And so I steamed each layer individually, hoping to restore the volume to the skirt, steaming from the inside, pulling on the fabric just like Marina taught me at *W* magazine.

Moments later, Grace appeared at my side like a phantom.

"Did you steam this dress?" she said, those eyes beating down on me.

"Yes," I said, my stomach turning over.

She got in close to my face. "You've breathed new life into that dress," she said. "I never thought it could look that way." She grabbed the dress off the rack and just as suddenly she was gone again.

When the shoot wrapped the next night, Grace, Mario Testino, Karen Elson, and a tight-knit group from their respective teams headed off to what we call a family dinner. Because that's the vibe on these sets; it takes a village to raise a fashion story. In a move of unheralded generosity, Grace thanked me for my hard work and invited me to join them to celebrate at Madeo, an Italian restaurant on Beverly.

I was floored. At dinner I sat across from Karen Elson, whom I idolized. She talked about her kids and Jack White and Nashville. And

Speak Up!

HOW TO START A CONVERSATION (EVEN WHEN YOU'RE TONGUE-TIED)

1. If you are shy, ask someone a question about themselves. It can be as simple as "How was your day today?"
2. Compliments always work! Try commenting on what someone is wearing, whether it be a piece of jewelry, a handbag, shoes, or a hairstyle.
3. If you can't speak, let your clothing talk for you. Wear something special that stands out in the crowd—an item of clothing or an accessory that you are extremely proud of. The way you are dressed can be a conversation starter. People will be complimenting you!

my only goal was to keep from being a creep. It was a very stylish crowd, and I couldn't believe I was sitting there. But I didn't want to sit there blinking. When people see me on television, they think that socializing comes naturally to me, that it's easy for me to be in a group. But I'm actually quite shy, and at dinner I had to force myself to participate in the conversation. Open your mouth! I told myself.

Everyone was enjoying the wine and Mario Testino kept talking about a party in the Hollywood Hills that we all *had to* go to. And Grace was ignoring phone calls from New York. I'd tested boundaries before, and I certainly wasn't going to drop in on a party in the Hills with Mario Testino. It was enough that I was invited to the dinner table. I didn't need to risk overstaying my welcome.

> "But I'm actually quite shy, and at dinner I had to force myself to participate in the conversation. Open your mouth! I told myself."

My Ten Favorite Fashion Icons*

*NOT INCLUDING THE OBVIOUS: MARILYN MONROE, MADONNA, AND GRACE CODDINGTON

1. Diana Ross
Think of her in Central Park singing in the rain in that red sequined jumpsuit. She's everything I like in a woman—feathers, sequins, flawless hair and makeup, and charm. And a little untouchable.

2. Courtney Love
Her baby-doll, grunge, Hole phase had a huge impact on me and my girlfriends. The nighties and baby barrettes and Mary Janes were so twisted and yet so genius.

3. Cary Grant
The classic gentleman. Whenever I want to dress handsome, without any trendy or super-fashionable overtones, I think, What would Cary Grant do?

4. Audrey Hepburn
Most people think of her in *Breakfast at Tiffany's,* but I love her in *Funny Face.* The black turtleneck, the ballet flats, the cropped pant—one of my favorite looks ever.

5. Molly Ringwald
I was—and still am—obsessed with John Hughes movies, and I loved her attitude. Wearing Ralph Lauren in *The Breakfast Club. Making* her prom dress in *Pretty in Pink.* The bridesmaid dress in *Sixteen Candles.* Three iconic fashion moments, all made successful by her attitude and mood.

6. Grace Kelly
Elegance, sophistication, and yes, grace.

7. Brad Pitt
He is the all-American guy but with European flair. He can do California beach but can also wear a beaded dress for the cover of *Rolling Stone*. He's modern and masculine, which isn't always easy to pull off. Plus, when I moved to Los Angeles, I dyed my hair blond to look like Brad in *Ocean's Eleven*.

8. Jackie O
The definition of chic.

9. James Dean
Casual ease but still grabs attention. He's also the inspiration for my hair.

10. Isabella Blow
She had the uncanny ability to know who or what would be the next big thing. Alexander McQueen, Philip Treacy, Julien Macdonald—she spotted them all first.

But I offered to drop off Mario and his two assistants at the party, because I was driving that way anyway. (And when Mario made a cell phone call to Kate Moss that night, I almost died.) Of course as soon as the valet pulled up with my car, I immediately regretted having volunteered. I looked in the backseat of my car and I could see all kinds of garbage on the floor. Items from my styling kit were spilled all over the backseat. I distinctly remember ducking into the backseat of the car to grab a pair of silicone boobs—chicken cutlets—and hide them.

"Don't mind these!" I said.

Despite the brush with Karen Elson and being in earshot of Kate Moss's cell phone calls, I had little to do with actual fashion at *Vogue*. I was fashion-world *adjacent*. If I'd been in New York full-time, walking around the halls of the mother ship, it might have been enough. But I wasn't so sure this was the right job for me. And I wondered where I was headed.

One afternoon an invitation arrived at the *Vogue* office, an invitation to a launch party for Rachel Zoe's style guide, *Style A to Zoe.* The party would be held on the roof of the Cartier store in Beverly Hills. I hadn't given up the dream of working for Rachel, and even though this invitation was addressed to Lisa Love, I RSVP'd for myself and put the invitation in my bag. It was a sin of omission. I wore short pants and a bow tie, basically a shrunken baby suit, and I went to the party alone. I planned on staying for one sparkling water, hoping to catch Rachel's attention. I wasn't even sure if she'd remember me. I saw her first, from across the room. We were at the Cartier store, and she looked like a Cartier watch. She was wearing a gold dress, vintage, and she not only remembered me but she seemed genuinely excited to see me.

"Come over here!" she shouted, intimating that I should hang out with her and her two assistants, Taylor and Leah, for the rest of the night. Minutes later, the four of us were dancing. I was as confused as you are. I was not alone in my confusion, by the way. Coincidentally, Candie— Gary's agent's wife, the one who brought me to that Chanel dinner with the backyard trains and the Picassos where I first met Rachel—was at the book party. When she spied me dancing with Rachel, she leaned in and said, "So, you're friends with her now?"

"I don't know!" I shouted over the music.

Later that night, I sat with Leah and told her all about my experience at *Vogue.* I was selling myself hard. I was name-dropping Mario Testino and Grace Coddington and saying how fabulous the job was. You better *werk*!

"Has Rachel hired anyone yet?" I said innocently.

"There might be a job open," Leah said.

When I left the party, Leah told me to expect a phone call.

. . . .

T here *was* a job open. And it was Leah's. This time, Rachel called herself. It was November when she filled me in on the specifics of the job—the hours, the salary, and what would be expected of me.

"That sounds amazing," I said.

But there is a little more to the story. What I didn't know was that Rachel was at work on a reality show, and Leah was leaving the company because she didn't want to be on television. I'd have to be involved in the reality show if I wanted the job. And shooting was to begin in January.

Um, OK. I had concerns. My first thought was, What is it going to look like? There aren't any fashion reality shows like this out yet. There was no established format. Even if there had been, I didn't know what "format" meant then. Yes, I'd be hands-on with clothing, which is what I didn't have at *Vogue*. Rachel addressed my hesitations head-on: "I'm an executive producer on it, so you know you're completely covered. I have the final say in everything. I'll never do anything against your will. I'll always have your back." She told me to call her in the next couple of days to give her an idea of where my head was at, and we hung up the phone. She'd need me as soon as possible, she said. If I decided to go with Rachel, I'd have to give my two weeks' notice immediately.

That night, I explained the situation to Gary. This was yet another not-quite-there moment in my life. Rachel Zoe was offering me my dream job. But if I wanted it, the trick was I had to agree to be on a major cable network show. Before Gary could get a word in I answered my own question: "I'm not interested," I said. Gary works in television, and he certainly understood. There were too many unknowns. We went to sleep. But sometime that night Gary had a change of heart. In the morning, he turned to me and said, "I was thinking about Rachel's offer. How are you going to feel if you watch that show and you know you were offered the chance to be her assistant?"

I thought about it. "I might feel like I missed out," I said. "I'll always be watching it and think, Maybe I should have given that a chance."

"I think you should consider it," he said. "If you're going to end up on a fashion reality show, you might as well end up on one with Rachel. She's always going to protect her image. She's not going to put out some shoddy product. How bad could it turn out to be?"

He had a point. But I still wasn't sold. I'd only been at *Vogue* for three months, and I was worried about burning bridges at the most important fashion magazine in the world. Besides, I hadn't even made it onto the masthead yet. And I was going to quit? I called my friend Annabet, who had worked for André Leon Talley at *Vogue* and successfully extricated herself to take a more senior position at *Jane* magazine. I was right to be concerned, she said. For all of the horror stories about *Vogue,* the magazine is a loyal place and a great nurturer of talent. There's this feeling: Once you're at *Vogue,* you're always at *Vogue.* It was like *The Godfather.* And I was turning my back on the family before I had a chance to make my mark.

There was more to the decision than just turning the page on the magazine. The more time I spent in fashion, the more I saw this great divide emerging: a bias between editorial stylists and celebrity stylists, a real church-and-state situation. You were either one or the other. That line in the sand would change in the coming years, thanks in large part to Rachel. Being a personal stylist would become a legitimate platform to mold and shape a vision and brand. It's less about red carpet moments than about giving a celebrity a real voice. But there was still that division. Should I continue on the *Vogue* path? Was that the better play? There was also my age to consider. I was thirty years old and I was an assistant. There was potential at the magazine, of course, great potential. But the path was well defined. Positions didn't open very often and I knew it would take quite a while for me to move up the ranks there. If I was twenty-three years old at the time, I wouldn't have even considered leaving. But I felt the clock ticking.

Project Runway

HOW TO DRESS FOR THE AIRPLANE. (HINT: DITCH THAT NECK PILLOW.)

Let's get this out of the way: I *can't* with the neck pillows and the sweat suits. Especially when you're traveling for work. You're going to be on a plane for four and a half hours. Why are you dressing like it's a pajama party? Dressing down for the airport is this weird phenomenon that's swept the nation. Suddenly you have to be in your most comfortable clothes to fly. OK, if you're on board a twelve-hour flight, fine. Bring a pair of sweatpants with you and change on the plane. But a four-hour flight to New York? Forget it. Also: Do those neck pillows even work? I don't know how wrapping your neck around a doughnut helps. But whatever.

There's this rumor I love about airplane travel: When Gisele Bündchen takes a flight, she sprays down her blanket and then the seat using essential oils so there's a pleasing smell. (Which I love.) I'm not saying you have to do that. But if you're flying to one of the most stylish cities in the world, it wouldn't hurt to put a little effort into your appearance.

Plan a travel outfit. How? Imagine you're going to brunch on Sunday with your best girlfriends. What would you wear? Maybe jeans and a cute little blazer and a striped T-shirt and a favorite bag? Maybe you'd bring a scarf for your neck, in case it got cold? Do the same on the plane. Think: What is an outfit you love that's not an evening dress?

If you're not willing to part with the in-flight sweat suit, do me (and the people around you) a favor: Pick one element. The top or the bottom. I sometimes wear a hoodie on the plane, because I like to cover my head when I sleep. But that hoodie, mind you, is Thom Browne.

You're on a plane, but you're still you. So wear a cute pair of jeans. Wear a nice pair of sneakers. Wear a pair of oxfords.

(CONTINUED ON NEXT PAGE)

Dress within your style. If you're taking an overnight flight, bring a change of clothes in your carry-on and get into the sweats on board. We're in the terminal eating dinner before the flight. I don't need to see what you sleep in. Speaking of which: Bring your own travel blanket. Those things in coach are *narsty*. Also, I don't mind if you bring your own food onto the plane. But please, no tuna fish sandwiches. We've gotta share this space, folks.

Last thing: That carry-on? Invest in something cute and functional. It can be a colorful tote, an overnight bag, a leather duffel, something vintage. But put some thought into it. Not everything has to be utilitarian. The whole idea of vacation is to relax and get away. These are milestones people look forward to all year while they're sitting in their cubicles. Why not be excited about the way you're going to look? Don't wear below-the-knee cargo shorts and shoes made for hiking Mt. Everest. A nice walking shoe will do.

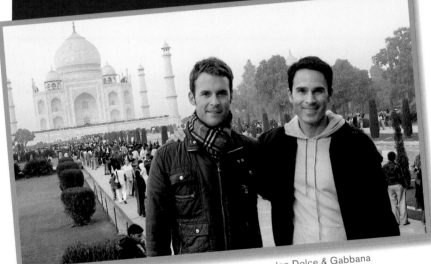

It's Christmas 2007 at the Taj Mahal, and I'm wearing a nylon Dolce & Gabbana motorcycle jacket—a present from Gary. The scarf is Burberry, and all together it's some effortless chic for the morning light in India. When you're being photographed in front of a landmark, you should wear something timeless.

All Aboard!

HOW TO PACK FOR A WEEKLONG VACATION IN TEN MINUTES

I often find myself at the airport checking in for a flight, standing behind a couple. A couple, as in two people. And yet they have six pieces of luggage. Meanwhile, the couple is dressed in sweatpants. I mean, what's inside all of those suitcases? More sweatpants?

When you're packing, lay out on the bed everything you'd like to bring with you. Then get out your itinerary and do an edit. If you're going to Hawaii or Mexico, figure you're going to spend more than half of your time at the beach or at the pool. Check the weather. Guys, bring at least two swimsuits. It's nice to switch it up. It's nice to have something to look forward to wearing the next day. Women, bring a variety of swimsuits. On a day when you're feeling good about your body and you want to get the most sun, wear a bikini. For the day when you feel like you ate too much the night before, you'll have a one-piece. Also, bring a variety of cover-ups. You'll be eating in them at the pool and they get dirty.

Side note: I don't have a problem with cover-ups when they're poolside. I do have a problem with people wearing bathing suits and cover-ups when they're in a restaurant or out shopping. Put on some shorts.

As for packing shoes, I am as guilty as the next guy, if not more so. I used to bring everything I owned on vacation. But everyone needs to calm down. You don't need eight pairs of shoes for one week. Look at the schedule. Think of how many nights you'll be going out. You'll be seen by people who've never met you. It's a good opportunity to let yourself shine. Once you get into the rhythm of your vacation, you'll wear two or three pairs of shoes. If you laid out four pairs of black shoes, put at least two back in

(CONTINUED ON NEXT PAGE)

the closet. You need a comfortable pair, a fashion day shoe—a fashion flat, a gladiator, or a day heel—and then for night, a party pump. Throw in a pair of flip-flops or an espadrille.

Comfortable doesn't mean lazy. It never does. A cute sundress can be just as effective as an evening gown. Pair it with a flat, and since you're on vacation, buy a pair of earrings to go with it.

When I go to the beach, I bring one jacket, just in case. I bring one or two pairs of light cotton pants—in a color if you're daring, khaki if not—though a pair of jeans is usually good enough. I bring two or three polo shirts and four T-shirts. I like to wear button-down shirts on the beach. They look cute with a swimsuit, blowing in the wind, pressing against your skin, teasing all of the boys.

The ultimate challenge: Try to limit yourself to just a carry-on bag. That's it. I don't roll my clothing. That doesn't work for me. I learned to fold during my days at the Gap. I fold it, then fold it in half. For years, I carried Prada luggage. Or, for a really quick trip, a Louis Vuitton bag or this bright red Bulgari. Now I'm into a roller carry-on from a German company called Rimowa. It's an investment. The bags are made from recycled World War II airplane parts, and they're indestructible. And the wheels rotate in different ways, so you can wheel it behind you or beside you.

If you're traveling in the summer and you can't fit everything into one nylon bag, you have a problem. I recently went on vacation to Europe for almost four weeks, and I traveled with one carry-on. I went on a cruise with my boyfriend that required formal wear—with only a carry-on. It can be done. You don't have to worry about your bag getting lost or waiting at the carousel. You can start your vacation thirty minutes earlier.

To allay my fears, Rachel set up a dinner for me and the producers of her nascent show. We went to Il Sole, a cozy Italian restaurant in West Hollywood, and Rachel was dripping in jewelry, dressed in some long-sleeved T-shirt thing down to her calves with a big fur vest over it. Her hair and makeup were flawless, and she had huge platform shoes and bell-bottoms on. The dinner was me, Rachel, Taylor, and Charlie Corwin, the executive producer of the show and the cofounder of Original Media. And, as if this whole thing wasn't awkward enough, sitting at the table next to us was one of Gary's best friends, who happened to be dining with Jodie Foster. Not only was I having dinner with Rachel Zoe, talking about a reality show we might do together and whether I should leave *Vogue*, I was trying not to stare at Clarice Starling.

I felt better but there was still a nagging feeling I couldn't shake. I needed a little more time to make a decision. Plus, I was preoccupied with two upcoming *Vogue* shoots, including one in Alaska that I'd leave for in two days.

"Go away on your shoots," Rachel said. "Take your time. But when you come back you should let me know your answer."

The night after dinner with Rachel, I found myself on the last flight to Kansas City and then on to Anchorage, courtesy of *Vogue*. We were hard at work on the magazine's upcoming Power Issue and a team had been dispatched from Los Angeles to the snowy reaches of the north to capture a then-unknown governor of Alaska at her home in Wasilla. This was my first major trip for the style bible I read as a kid growing up in Canada. While I was under immense pressure, I realized this was one of those rare moments in life when one is exactly where one wants to be. Except in my fashion daydreams I never once imagined I might die a frozen death on the side of a highway—in a red state, no less.

The conditions there were treacherous. And I'm just talking about the roads. We hadn't even *met* the governor's team yet, though they'd been quite vocal in phone calls. ("Sarah Palin will not be photographed without her glasses," they'd repeated.) I was in the backseat of a black SUV surrounded by photo equipment and garment bags on a two-hour drive from Anchorage to the mountainside, log-cabin bed-and-breakfast where we'd set up our fashion base camp. There were no lights on the highway and the driver was swerving wildly. On three distinct occasions I was sure we were about to tumble off the road. I am not a professional driver, but having grown up in wintry Ontario I know for certain that slamming on the brakes in a skid is a big no-no. This is the life of a fashion assistant, and it was something I'd need to get used to if I was going to work for Rachel.

Somehow, we made it to Wasilla in time for a late-night dinner at what we'd been assured was the best restaurant in town. Because we were in Alaska, I was expecting fresh king crab legs and wild king salmon. Instead, we were served thawed flounder on a bed of frozen peas and rice pilaf; the salad was three leaves of iceberg lettuce with shredded carrot on top. I'm sad to report the provisions were not much better the next morning in Sarah Palin's living room, where we were served homemade moose-meat sausage. I know we were in Wasilla and all. But seriously: Who serves homemade moose sausage to a crew from *Vogue*?

As an assistant, it was my job to unpack all of the trunks and set up the racks of clothing so the editor could have it all laid out before her. Though we were traveling with twelve trunks, on a shoot like this, inevitably the fashion editor will decide something is missing and the whole operation will fall apart if we can't immediately find this one particular pair of shoes. This shoot was, of course, no exception. I'd arranged something like a hundred pairs of shoes and boots in the Palin family room when my editor asked, "Where are the Sorel boots?"

Uh-oh.

It's one thing if you're at a photo studio in Los Angeles when you discover a particular brand of furry boot is missing. Even if it's a particular model of furry boot not yet in the stores, that's still a problem that's easily solved. It's only slightly more complicated when you're in the backwoods of Wasilla. Still, I sprang into action and got on the phone with an assistant in our New York office.

"Do you have the Sorel boots?"

"Yes," the frightened voice said.

Great. But how to get them to Alaska, gulp, *today*? I made a phone call to the Worldnet courier service. And after being placed on hold, I found out that—for more money than Todd Palin probably spent on the snowmobile parked in the driveway—we could have these magic boots airlifted directly to the Palin residence by same-day express.

"Should we spend the money?" I asked the editor. Actually, that's a joke. Of course we'd spend the money. Child, it's *Vogue*!

Sarah Palin, meanwhile, was in hair and makeup, being painted by the professionals we'd brought in. Though I had never heard this woman's name before this trip, it was clear even then that she had bigger aspirations. Because she was into the *Vogue* makeover, big-time. I was steaming dresses in earshot of the makeup chair when Palin's mother appeared over her shoulder.

"You look beautiful," she said.

Palin looked at herself in the mirror and had to agree with her mom, speaking like only an Alaskan can. "It's better than having moose blood sprayed across my face!" Palin said.

By the way, miracles did happen. The glasses came off. We got our shot—and it was beautiful. She looked fantastic, and the Alaskan landscape did not disappoint. It is a beautiful place. And those Sorel boots finally arrived from New York in time, though once the fur-and-leather shoes were unpacked and seen in the flesh, the editor decided they weren't necessary after all. Oh, well. We got our shot. And just as suddenly, I was on a flight out, exhausted but proud of myself and my work, feeling that I'd not only passed this test but earned some serious stripes. I proved to myself and my boss—and to Sarah Palin—that I belonged in this world.

And to belong was all I ever wanted. It's all anyone can ask for in this life, really. For me, it was fashion that first made me think this was possible. Or that *more* was possible.

And more was possible for me. I'd made my decision. In a way, my training at *Vogue* was perfect preparation for life with Rachel: It was the beginning of my being whisked away to far-flung locations and praying that boxes show up.

I sent Rachel an e-mail: "I'm in Alaska, standing on a frozen lake in a Balenciaga shearling aviator jacket, and I wanted to let you know that I'm going to take the job."

> "In a way, my training at *Vogue* was perfect preparation for life with Rachel: It was the beginning of my being whisked away to far-flung locations and praying that boxes show up."

7

It's OK to cry. Just not on the red carpet.

WORKING FOR RACHEL ZOE was dramatic from day one. Actually, it was dramatic from *before* day one. Let me explain: Gary and I were on vacation in St. Barts for New Year's Eve. It was December 2007, and by chance, Rachel and her husband, Rodger, were also in St. Barts. Rachel invited us to have a drink at her hotel—a sort of welcome-to-the-team toast. But I realized there was more to this meeting than a simple celebratory clink when I sat down and Rachel mentioned a last-minute job she'd just accepted styling Brad Pitt for a Japanese cell phone company, SoftBank. She politely asked-slash-suggested I fly home early from my vacation to start pulling clothes for the job.

The weather in St. Barts was perfect. But the truth was, I was happy to go. This is what it means to be an assistant. Your life is not your own. That family vacation you think you're taking? That trip with your boyfriend? Forget it. Everything is tentative. You're subject to the whims of your boss's schedule *and* the client's schedule. Yes, these jobs promise a view into a glamorous world and you'll be surrounded by beautiful people and more beautiful clothing, but it comes with a price, and that price is sacrificing your calendar and sometimes your relationships. You need to know that up front. I was happy to do it. I was there to learn. And it began.

This was my dream job, and I was all in. At the time, Rachel was working out of her home studio, a white-walled garage tacked at the front of her midcentury-modern house in the Hollywood Hills. The floors were concrete, and the room was full of rolling racks. I showed up on that first day and let myself in. Taylor had her back to me, and she barely turned around to acknowledge my existence.

"This is so pointless," she said. "There's no reason for you to be back here." It was quite an introduction. My dream was to work for Rachel, but for the first few days, Taylor was my boss. I tried to remember this was a transition for her, too. She and my predecessor, Leah, had been best friends. Taylor wasn't unkind to me. She wasn't frustrated with me. She was frustrated to be back at work.

And I can't exactly blame her. It was Wednesday, January 2, 2008—not quite a holiday in Los Angeles but the fashion showrooms and the PR agencies were all closed. We were supposed to be calling in clothing for Brad Pitt, but there was very little to do except make lists of people we planned on calling once the stores reopened. It was just Taylor and me in a garage with clothing racks. There was no new-job orientation. There was no employee training.

And by the way, I needed it! Very early on—like, on the first day—I realized that I had no business working for Rachel Zoe. She'd hired me, in large part, because I worked at *Vogue,* and I was sure she liked how that sounded. While I could call in clothing and I knew how to act on set, I had a lot to learn. I didn't really know how to set up a fitting or how to get a tailor. I had the PR list from *Vogue,* but I was essentially cold-calling the fashion houses to request garments for Rachel's clients. No one knew me. They had no reason to.

There were some early hiccups. Taylor asked me to send some clothing back to some designers, but she gave me the wrong FedEx number. She had inadvertently transposed two digits. I copied that number onto thirty FedEx slips, and all of these packages were charged to some random account. Once FedEx figured out the mistake, I spent a full day reversing the charges.

Somehow, by the time Rachel flew home from St. Barts, we'd pulled twelve racks of clothing together for the Brad Pitt shoot, including pieces from Tom Ford and Burberry, plus tons of vintage motorcycle jackets and vintage T-shirts from What Goes Around Comes Around, a great resource in New York and L.A. for hard-to-find pieces. We'd filled the studio, with four additional racks spilling over into the hallway, and Rachel seemed happy.

The Brad Pitt shoot was scheduled for Hollywood Studios on Gower, in the center of Hollywood. And the vibe fit Brad perfectly: He has that aura that certain super-famous people have, like a special force field is glowing around them. His perfection is mind-blowing. He doesn't seem human, but yet seems so human at the same time. He was wonderfully polite, though, as he went through the racks, and he actually wanted to purchase a lot of the clothing for himself, which felt like a victory. Though for the mobile phone commercial itself—for the job we'd been hired to do—he wore his own boots and jeans, the ones he showed up in that morning. From the twelve racks of clothing we pulled, he ended up wearing one T-shirt and one vintage motorcycle jacket. That's it.

Meanwhile, I spent most of the shoot in a side room with Taylor, eating hors d'oeuvres, pot stickers, spring rolls, and sliders from the catering table. It was the antithesis of anything Grace Coddington preached. I worried that I was like that guy in the Dickies pants whom Grace yelled at for treating catering like a horse trough.

This turned out to be the calm before the storm.

We started filming the first season of *The Rachel Zoe Project* only one week after I arrived, and none of us had a clue how it would work. I showed up in the morning and a production assistant slapped a microphone on me, and then I went about my day pretending there wasn't a camera in my face or incredibly bright lighting overhead. The producers hung out in the studio for hours just waiting for something—anything, really—to happen. Taylor, God love her, was a pain in the ass to the crew from the very beginning. On camera, she taunted the producers, saying ridiculous things like "This is the most boring show ever. Nobody is going to watch this."

As for me, I was more concerned with learning the job than with the cameras. Unfortunately, my responsibilities were never clearly defined. This was a real job for me but nobody was telling me what to do. I felt lost more often than not. I styled Kate Beckinsale for some press she was doing for an indie called *Snow Angels*. And when I came home at night to Gary, I locked myself in the home office and cried. I was seventeen again. It was sink or swim, and I was worried that Taylor might let me sink. Our personalities didn't mesh. She liked to get the job done and get home. I was the opposite. I wanted to stay and hang out with Rachel and ask questions and be chatty and get to know her and find out how things worked there. This was the extent of what I knew: Rachel had an enviable client list, and Taylor and I were each to run point on certain accounts. Taylor worked closely with Jennifer Garner, Eva Mendes, and Cameron Diaz. And I was to work with Kate Beckinsale and Joy Bryant. (Later, when Anne Hathaway came aboard, I'd work with her, too.)

I had been working for Rachel for three weeks when we flew to New York for Fashion Week. My eyes were beyond wide. I'd never done a proper Fashion Week, only crashed events when I could beg my way in. Now I was staying at a gorgeous hotel and had a packet of tickets with my name on them. I thought I'd be standing in the back, at best, but at most of these shows I was seated directly behind Rachel. The *Rachel Zoe Project* crew was following us around, and it was madness. The Waverly Inn was the restaurant of the season. We ate there three or four times that week. Francisco Costa from Calvin Klein was at one table. Oscar de la Renta and Valentino were at another table. I was getting whiplash looking around the room. Rachel introduced me to Valentino and the only thought in my head was, I'm so glad I didn't eat today. Because I'm so nervous I could throw up right now. We had dinner with Brian Atwood and Nate Berkus, and I ordered the chicken pot pie and the biscuits and the berry crumble. Thom Browne was at the next table and I was speechless.

> "I was seventeen again. It was sink or swim, and I was worried that Taylor might let me sink."

When I thought the insanity couldn't get any more intense, a phone call came and my itinerary changed wildly. While I couldn't be trusted to change the toner in the office copy machine, I was about to be handed my first major international assignment, and the stakes were stiletto-high. This trip would determine my standing with the top celebrity stylist in the country, and perhaps my future in fashion.

> "I was about to be handed my first major international assignment, and the stakes were stiletto-high."

My phone pinged at two in the morning with a text: "911." I thought it was a joke. But Rachel said: "We need to get an entire fitting together today for an international press tour for Kate Hudson."

Fashion Week is all about scouting dresses for the upcoming awards season, but now Kate Hudson had dropped a fashion emergency in our laps. The in-demand actress was about to leave town for the BAFTA Awards in London when she had a last-minute crisis of faith. She wanted to change her look, and that meant changing her stylist and bringing Team Zoe in. Kate was scheduled to depart for Europe in less than forty-eight hours and she needed a dress for the awards ceremony, plus looks for the Elle Style Awards in the UK and for a round of interviews with the media. Could we pull a fitting together on a moment's notice? Oh, and could I go to London with her?

Though I was in runway shows with Rachel all day on the lookout for Oscar dresses, I threw up the fashion equivalent of the Bat Signal, asking publicists to send over anything that might work for Kate. Taylor had already gone home to L.A., and this was one of the first jobs I was really handling on my own. From my seat in the shows, I was e-mailing publicists at the different fashion houses requesting looks for Kate to wear in London. I was in the car e-mailing. I was on the toilet e-mailing. I was running from show to show, praying that when I got back to the hotel for that night's fitting, the right clothing would be there waiting for me. I thought back on my time at *W* magazine and how stressed Marina had been. Finally, I got it. I never realized how much energy and hustle it took to pull something like this together.

> **"I never realized how much energy and hustle it took to pull something like this together.... I lived for the stress because I was so fresh."**

I wasn't scared of Rachel. I was just afraid of disappointing her. She set the expectations high and pushed you to be a better assistant, to work at a certain level. I lived for the stress because I was so fresh.

Garment bags started arriving around noon and continued through the evening. It was all on the line for me, and I had planned for every possible contingency. Kate showed up that night and was thankfully happy with the looks. I'd pulled off a last-minute fitting at the height of Fashion Week. I was out to prove that I was more than just the guy in the bow tie who is fun to have around. That I could do this job. That I could be trusted with an A-list client. Because if I couldn't cut it, there were a million girls waiting to take my place. Which is just one of the many ways the fashion world is like *Showgirls*. Like the poster says, "Leave your inhibitions at the door."

Suddenly I was in London, surrounded by racks of clothing and a minibar stocked with Toblerone up to my arms. It was a terrible time to come down with the flu, but that is exactly what happened. After a thirty-six-hour incubation period, a tickle in the back of my throat had blossomed into a head-to-toe fever, and I was unable to lift my head off the pillow. While I tried to kill the bug by sleeping it off, there are some things even six-hundred-thread-count sheets can't fix. I woke up in a puddle of my own sweat, at which point three thoughts went through my head, not necessarily in this order:

> "I was out to prove that I was more than just the guy in the bow tie who is fun to have around. That I could do this job. That I could be trusted with an A-list client."

1. If I don't get out of bed, I'm going to get fired from my dream job before it even begins.
2. Do hotels still have doctors on call?
3. I really wish *The Devil Wears Prada* was on TV.

Also, a fourth question: How exactly did I get here?

I asked myself that question all the time. Our schedules changed that often and without warning. Three days ago I had been asleep in New York at another boutique hotel. Now I was plagued by something resembling the Black Death, and I had to force myself to put on a brave face as I readied Kate for the awards ceremony. In the end, it wasn't the flu that threatened to sink my styling career. It was the zipper on a taffeta Valentino gown.

I learned an invaluable lesson on this trip—and it isn't that London hotels no longer have doctors on call (though that is also good to know). As a stylist, you can have the best eye in the world, but that eye will only get you so far. What you need to be is a good salesperson. In New York, Kate had chosen a strapless, red Valentino gown, tight to mid-calf. But after two hours of hair and makeup in London, she slid into this perfect dress only to see the zipper go off the track. Full-blown panic, right? Not a chance.

> "As a stylist, you can have the best eye in the world, but that eye will only get you so far. What you need to be is a good salesperson."

It was time to put on my salesman hat. We got her out of the Valentino and I started pushing Dress B—a gold, sequined Dior gown with a low back. It was very art deco looking, and it went perfectly with a pair of diamond-and-emerald Bulgari shower earrings we'd picked out.

This broken zipper was a happy accident, I told her. And I believed that: In a way, the best dress really did win in the end. And she looked gorgeous. The fashion blogs went crazy for the look—and then flipped again a few nights later for her look at the Elle Style Awards. Kate looked gorgeous in a white keyhole Derek Lam—with a 1970s door knocker vintage Van Cleef necklace for a Studio 54 moment. That was a double victory: On top of looking stunning, wearing Derek Lam allowed her to endorse a fashion-world rising star. When a major Hollywood star chooses to wear an up-and-coming New York designer to a big international fashion event she's making a statement. This was a chance for Kate to use her voice. She is a fashion icon, and she is rewarded for taking risks.

In the end, the Valentino zipper was repaired in New York. Kate was

Power Up!

HOW TO KEEP YOUR ENERGY HIGH WHEN YOU'RE ON THE GO

1. Get to bed! Trust me, I have my fair share of sleepless nights or nights when I arrive home from a party at four A.M. It's important to get at least six hours of sleep. No excuses.
2. If you are tired, don't talk about how tired you are. I believe that manifests more exhaustion. Be extra kind to yourself and the world on these days.
3. Drink lots of water. Caffeine is delicious and will keep you up, but staying hydrated is more important.
4. Exercise is key—even when you're tired. Push yourself.
5. Eat a real meal. Eating on the go is necessary at times, but sit for fifteen minutes, put down your iPhone, and enjoy your meal. Carry some snacks with you, too. I get so crazy when my blood sugar is too low. Keep a nutrition bar or some nuts on hand to help you get through to your next meal. Or stop to get a juice or a smoothie—my favorite fix when I feel my energy lagging.

happy. As for me, I nursed a fever on a thirteen-hour flight to Los Angeles, fighting off the chills. But I was proud of myself and felt like I was making real progress with Rachel. That I'd established myself as a reliable second assistant. Or so I thought.

Let me start here: From the outset, Rachel and I were best girlfriends. We'd go through look books together. We'd talk about our favorite models. We loved to see the clothing in real life—that was the real thrill of this job. To touch the clothing. We discussed what we were going to wear to the office every day, and she quickly became my first call of the day and my last text at night. On national television, Taylor would accuse me of being "up Rachel's ass." And I kinda was.

Rachel was like a Barbie doll come to life. She looked like Barbie.

Bringing Sexy Back

OR WHAT YOU CAN LEARN FROM MARILYN MONROE

One of the first things I noticed in Los Angeles was a confusion among people about what is sexy. A minidress and platform heels and tons of makeup and hair—I'm all for that moment. But there's something to be said for how sexy a bit of subtle sophistication can be. It's important to remember: Don't give it all away. Rely on the element of surprise. There's a great power in undressing and revealing what's been hidden.

There's a little bit of the burlesque dancer in me, and it comes out in styling. I like to reveal things slowly. Madonna pushed boundaries and got everything right. But that doesn't mean everyone should wear a cone bra. A semi-sheer blouse with a great bra and a pencil skirt can be more effective. There's a way of showing off your body without giving it all away that can be much more appealing. In styling Jessica Alba, I channel Maria Callas, Sophia Loren. For the CFDA Awards, I took inspiration from a 1970s yacht in Saint-Tropez. It's about characters and imagination.

This very much extends to men. There's nothing worse than a man in a skintight T-shirt with a waxed chest and embroidered pockets on his jeans and a horrible square-toed Italian shoe. Men in Italy don't dress this way. Have you been to Rome? What they do so well there is the perfectly tailored suit with a crisp white shirt open to reveal a little bit of chest. That's sexy. And there are a thousand men like that in Rome walking out their doors every morning.

You don't need to spend a lot of money, either, if you know your shape. You can buy a suit for $200, as long as you take it to a tailor and spend an extra $75 to have it fit your body. You don't need fifty suits in your closet. You need six: charcoal, navy, and khaki in winter and summer weights. Have the bases covered.

Take a lesson from Marilyn Monroe. She was sexy but she never gave it all away.

She had a never-ending closet of amazing clothing. I'd get to dress her up just like I'd done with my dolls. It was like a childhood fantasy come to life. More than that, we had a fashion mind-meld. We were in synch. At runway shows, I'd sit behind her furiously trading e-mails. I'd be e-mailing the head of Chanel PR from the third row as looks were coming down the runway. When the look books came out, Rachel and I had the same thoughts. She'd say, "Did you see look number forty-three? That's so Cameron." And because I'd felt the same way, I'd already e-mailed the publicist to request the look. It was one big fashion game. How many looks could I call in that Rachel wanted?

It was everything I'd hoped and wished for. And yet, when I was pushed, I contemplated walking away. Allow me to present the Case of Oscar Week 2008.

It was February 2008 and Rachel's studio was a whirlwind of activity. Boxes were arriving from Zac Posen, Armani, and Dior. We did a shoot with the Japanese model Jessica Michibata, who has been called Japan's answer to Gisele Bündchen. I felt like I was in *Lost in Translation*. We had the Art of Elysium benefit, the SAG Awards, plus Rachel was styling two *Details* covers—with Ashton Kutcher and Christian Bale. There were never less than four or five racks of clothing coming and going from the office at any moment. And I was just trying to keep up. Not to mention that there was a camera crew following us. And tensions were rising between me and Taylor. She talked to me like I was a child. She ranted to the camera, "He's never available to help me. I shouldn't be unpacking boxes." I relied on the tools I learned in AA. *One day at a time. Restraint of tongue and pen.* If I'd unleashed everything I wanted to say, I would have been fired. But if you're going to get sober, you can't act like you did when you were drunk in sober situations. And so I took the abuse, even when it was without merit. I could not change Taylor. But I could change my reaction to her.

Rachel had two clients presenting at the Oscars plus five others attending parties. It was a dozen fittings and clothing pulls to get through the week.

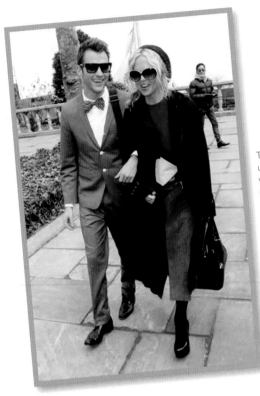

This picture sums up my relationship with Rachel—two girlfriends walking through Bryant Park during Fashion Week.

We had the Independent Spirit Awards, too, and when Rachel said, "There's no margin for error. The entire world is watching," she wasn't kidding.

For the fashion world, the Oscar season begins in January with the couture collections. We're trying to get the best looks for our clients. But there are so many premieres and press days over the season that dresses disappear fast. Millions of people watch the Oscars, and those photos run forever. It's become more of a fashion show than an awards show, and there is so much pressure to get it right. Everyone knows who styles each of these major stars. And if someone isn't known, and a starlet pulls off a major red carpet moment, believe me, the next day you'll know the name of the stylist who pulled it all together. The days of wearing a Gap shirt with a Vera Wang ball gown—as Sharon Stone did in the nineties—are disappearing.

Oscar day was all about dividing and conquering. Taylor was scheduled to help Cameron Diaz get ready while I went to Kate Beckinsale's house to get her dressed for Elton John's annual Oscar party with *InStyle*. The pressure was mounting and there were nights when I woke up in a cold sweat screaming. It was like going into battle, and we needed reinforcements. Taylor and I went shopping for our kits: our superhero fashion tool belts, stocked with everything you might need in a styling emergency, including shoe pads, nipple covers, Topstick tape, a steamer, an assortment of bras and underwear, stain remover, a mini sewing kit. We stopped by a lingerie store, Under G's, for nipple covers.

Suddenly it was February 24, 2008, Oscar Sunday. In international news, Fidel Castro announced his retirement that day. But I had my own Cuban missile crisis on my hands when I found out that the plans were changing: I was going to be dressing Cameron Diaz that afternoon. Keep in mind that I barely knew her. And she's one of the biggest movie stars in the world. I met her exactly once. I didn't know what accessories she'd looked at, or what shoes she'd tried on, or what clutch she was going to carry. But due to some scheduling changes, Taylor needed to be with Jennifer Garner and I was dispatched to take care of Cameron Diaz.

"What am I supposed to bring?" I asked Taylor, and she pointed to two pairs of shoes.

"Did you guys actually confirm shoes for Cameron? I'm nervous there's only two pairs."

Taylor: "Yeah."

Me: "So I don't need to stick more in here?"

Taylor: "No."

I blame myself. I should have known better. I'd only been working for Rachel for six weeks. But if nothing else, I knew that Rachel loved having options at the ready. For standard red carpet events, we *always* had at least two rows of shoes. An outfit is never really decided or confirmed until a client physically walks out the door. There were at least fifteen bags laid out on the bed. Not to mention the jewelry. Cartier, Van Cleef, Bulgari. No matter what happened in a fitting, there was always a gray area, and we were expected to be prepared. And yet! This was the Oscars, the biggest fashion day of the year, and all I was supposed to bring to Cameron Diaz was two pairs of shoes and one bag? OK . . .

So there I was in a suite at the Sunset Marquis in West Hollywood preparing for Cameron Diaz's arrival. I set the clutch out on the bed and arranged the two pairs of heels Taylor had told me to bring. The dress, a gorgeous pink Dior gown by John Galliano, was hanging in the closet. I set the jewelry out, including a white gold and diamond ring from Bulgari, plus Van Cleef and Cartier. That's it. Rachel and I barely spoke that morning. The only bit of instruction she gave me was to have Cameron look at the jewelry, then set aside what she liked and have the rest sent away.

Cameron Diaz showed up. She pulled two sets of Bulgari jewelry from the pieces on the counter, and I packed up the rest. I figured, at this point, she's Cameron Diaz. Who is going to tell her what jewelry to wear? She can wear whatever she feels comfortable in. So I smiled. I told her she looked gorgeous (and she did—like a goddess). I gave her a kiss on the cheek, sent the rest of the jewels away, and headed over to Kate Beckinsale's house way up in the Palisades to help her get ready for the Elton John party. Unfortunately, when I arrived she was having second thoughts about the jewelry we confirmed in her fitting. She loved the dress, a brown Versace Atelier gown, but it was still hanging on a rack. Her daughter was coloring in the living room.

"I'll figure this out," I said, trying to sound calm. It's important to maintain a sense of control in front of a client. But once I was out of earshot, I fell apart. It was the day of the Oscars, I was standing in Kate's guest room with no cell phone reception, and I was frantically trying to call the publicists at Van Cleef and Cartier to pull a diamond-encrusted rabbit out of a hat. "Bring everything you have left up to the house," I said. And they did. This is reason number one that you have to be kind to people and develop good relationships. Because on the day everyone in the fashion world is stretched beyond thin, you're going to need a favor. You'll need four armed guards to come up to a beautiful woman's house to hand-deliver new jewelry options.

I was stressing out when my BlackBerry somehow pulled a signal from the sky and started blowing up with a backlog of text messages from Taylor and then from Rachel herself. *Ping ping ping.*

From Taylor, the messages read something like this:

"Where are you?"

"Pick up."

"You're in so much trouble."

"WHERE ARE THE COATS FOR DEMI!"

Oh, boy. OK. Now that one was my fault. Demi Moore and Madonna were cohosting a last-minute, top-secret Oscar party at Guy Oseary's house in Beverly Hills. And Taylor had asked me to pull some coats and drop them off at Demi's house along with the dress we'd arranged for her to wear. I dropped off the dress, but I completely forgot to pull any jackets, and so Taylor had to do it herself.

I was driving down the hill from Kate's—sweating through my Michael Kors black cashmere hoodie and my Rag & Bone riding blazer—when I finally had enough cell reception to call Taylor. "You really screwed up," she says. "This is not good. We're all waiting for you here at the house." Apparently, there had been more mayhem: Rachel was with Cameron Diaz at the Sunset Marquis, and she didn't have a styling kit with her. And it was my fault. Apparently I was supposed to have built a kit for her and left it behind at the hotel. Except no one told me to do this. Not only was Rachel freaking out because she didn't have a kit but she also didn't have enough jewelry to play with. When Rachel couldn't reach me on the phone, she called her makeup artist, Joey, in a panic, and he rushed over to the Sunset Marquis with some styling supplies. By the time my phone got any reception, Cameron was already safely dressed in Dior and on her way to the red carpet. But not without a final emergency: She was in desperate need of a shoe pad, and Rachel didn't have one in Joey's makeshift kit. So Cameron had to fashion one herself, MacGyver style, tearing the insole from another shoe and pushing it into the new heels.

I was on my way to Rachel's when I called Gary, who told me to pull over to the side of the road. I was hyperventilating and he couldn't understand a word I was saying and he was convinced I was going to get in an accident. There I was, on the side of Sunset Boulevard on Oscar Sunday, having a panic attack while Gary tried to talk me off the ledge. "Pull yourself together," he said. "Go back to the house. Listen to what they have to say. But whatever you do, don't cry. Because if they're filming and you cry you'll regret it."

Of course Gary was right. I pulled up to Rachel's house and a sound guy from *The Rachel Zoe Project* tried to put a microphone pack on me.

"I don't want to be mic'd," I said.

Yeah, right. This was clearly going to be the grand finale of the first season. I walked into the studio and Taylor was there, ready to pounce. I made a beeline to Rachel's guest bedroom, where I sat with her and apologized. Taylor, meanwhile, was screaming at me through the wall. "You didn't get coats for Demi! Stop protecting him!" I was partially to blame. But it got so heated that Rachel was now consoling *me*.

"Common sense is leaving a kit!" Taylor shouted.

No, common sense is when you see someone upset, you don't freak out on them. You talk to them in a human way. I turned to Rachel and said, "I'm done. I quit. I'm not coming back." And I believed it. I'd been working with her for six weeks. This was my dream job, but there were major gaps in the information I was getting. I couldn't do my job this way, let alone learn anything—which was the point of all of this.

And the Winner Is . . .

THE TEN BEST OSCAR LOOKS EVER (IN NO PARTICULAR ORDER)

Julia Roberts (2001), vintage Valentino

Black-and-white is always the go-to for instant chic. It's so closely associated with Chanel and the French elite. But black-and-white can also be a bit boring. There are other pitfalls here: I love vintage, but a vintage gown can lose its modernity. But I remember seeing Julia on the carpet in this vintage Valentino and thinking, If I was going to win an Oscar, this is the way I'd want to look. No one has been able to do black-and-white truly right since. Julia isn't known for her red carpet style, necessarily. But this *Erin Brockovich* moment was the one time that counted for her on the red carpet, and she stole the show.

Hilary Swank (2005), Guy Laroche

From the front, Hilary Swank was basically in a navy blue burka. But when she turned around it was like the gasp heard around the world. The dress was backless down to, oh, just above her butt crack. It was an example of giving a lot away, but at the same time not giving anything away. Swank had some bubblegum-pink tutu madness moment a few years before. But this Guy Laroche dress was a million-dollar comeback for the *Million Dollar Baby.*

Audrey Hepburn (1954), Givenchy

This is one of those iconic dresses that everyone references. It's a boatneck gown with the kind of heavy corset construction that dreams are made of. That waist? What is that, twenty-three inches? The proportions of her body and the shoulder and the waist and the full skirt are something that I *actually* dream about. I wonder if it might be hard to get the attention of the press today

(CONTINUED ON NEXT PAGE)

with such an understated choice. But this look embodies the elegance and sophistication that Audrey Hepburn represents.

Michelle Williams (2006), Vera Wang

There hadn't been a lot of color on the red carpet in recent years, but then Michelle Williams—nominated for *Brokeback Mountain*—turned up in a canary-yellow Vera Wang with a plunging tulle neckline and Chopard diamonds. The red lip, the perfect blond hair. I hate the term "old Hollywood glamour," but sometimes it's called for.

Farrah Fawcett (1978), Stephen Burrows

This is the seventies at its best. Gold mesh and barely covering her breasts, this dress gave you the illusion that you'd get a peek at something. Farrah remained true to her style, but in a sophisticated, event-appropriate way. This is 1970s disco at the Oscars, and it was perfection.

Anne Hathaway (2009), Armani Privé

Full disclosure: I was involved in this look. But that's not why I chose it. This was the first dress Anne tried on, and we knew this would be the dress. We spent two weeks fitting other gowns, just to be sure. But she needed the Armani Privé—which was couture, beautifully made, strapless with sequins set diagonally. It was a big year for her. It was her first nomination, for *Rachel Getting Married*, and this was the right amount of glitz and glamour, without invoking Liza Minnelli.

Marion Cotillard (2008), Jean Paul Gaultier Couture

Talk about a risk. Jean Paul Gaultier's entire collection that year was based on the sea—with fish scales and mermaids on everything. For Marion, this look was a combination of so many things that could have gone wrong: white, fish scales, rosettes around the boobs, and a ton of beading. It could have looked like a bad costume from a Bette Midler show. But because Marion wears clothes so well and doesn't let the clothing wear her, her look is effortless. Even though the dress was nothing *but* effort. Plus, for a French actress to wear a French designer on this major night in her career was a nice nod to where she's from.

Penélope Cruz (2007), Atelier Versace
Before she played a fiery artist in *Vicky Cristina Barcelona*, Penélope Cruz was bringing serious drama to the red carpet. Then she was nominated for her role in *Volver*. As a stylist and as a viewer, this is one of those big moments that you're waiting for. She's this tiny girl in an awfully big ruffled gown, with perfect hair, makeup, and jewelry. She was a fantasy come to life.

Sharon Stone (1999), Vera Wang
Talk about DIY. It takes a confident, assured woman—or maybe it takes balls—to go into her husband's closet, grab a Gap shirt, and wear it to the Oscars. End of story.

Nicole Kidman (1997), Christian Dior Couture
Let's start with the color: chartreuse. Add on that deep burgundy lip, the Indian jewelry, and the shape of her body in this sleeveless gown with a hint of fur trim. Do you know how beautiful this gown was? So beautiful that everybody forgot Tom Cruise was standing next to her.

"Don't quit," Rachel said. "We'll figure it out."

"I don't want to figure it out. I'm going to have pizza with my boyfriend." I picked up my keys, took off my microphone pack, and walked out the front door. On the way to Farfalla pizza on Hillhurst, I called my sister from the car. "Taylor is bad news," she said. "You're never going to win. You should get out of there."

I was driving home with the pizza when my phone started ringing.

I looked down and saw Taylor's name pop up on the screen. I ignored her call. Then I ignored her second call. Finally I picked up. I knew this conversation would be recorded for the show, that the cameras at Rachel's house would be getting all of this on video. But I picked up anyway. Because I knew Taylor wouldn't stop calling if I didn't answer.

"Don't quit," Taylor said. "Come back in. We'll work things out."

I wasn't so sure. Everything I feared was coming true. I felt sabotaged. But worse, I felt like taking this job had been a mistake. I was a grunt at *Vogue*, but at least I was a grunt at the world's most important fashion magazine. When I quit after only three months, I was told I'd be blacklisted from Condé Nast. At the time, a photographer told me, "Fuck them." He said, "The second you become successful and make a name for yourself, those magazines will come sniffing around you. Do what you need to do." But maybe this had all been a mistake, a rash panic move. I'd given up all credibility and my career trajectory to be on some TV show, and though I hadn't seen any of the footage yet, I certainly knew how I'd be perceived—which is to say, like an incompetent queen. I'd let a twenty-four-year-old blond girl from Beverly Hills walk all over me, and to make matters worse, I cried about it on camera. And I cried ugly.

> "I'd given up all credibility and my career trajectory to be on some TV show, and though I hadn't seen any of the footage yet, I certainly knew how I'd be perceived."

When I got home, Gary was sympathetic. But he was also a realist.

"Did you cry?" he asked.

"Yes."

"Well, get ready to see that in every promo."

8

If you're not making mistakes, you're not growing.

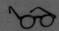

THE RACHEL ZOE PROJECT premiered on September 8, 2008, becoming a cult hit for Bravo. Looking at the TV show each week, I was able to see the events with some distance. I could see just how far I came in such a short time and how much I learned from Rachel and Taylor. And I am so glad that I took Gary's advice, that I looked at this opportunity and went for it. Because Gary was right: If I'd turned on this show and seen this positive outpouring of love and these insane opportunities directed at some other aspiring stylist, I would have felt like I'd missed out. It was scary to leave *Vogue*. But sometimes you have to leave one amazing opportunity to pursue

another, to find out what you can do. What I was discovering was that I
was much more than the kid who forgot to leave a kit for Rachel.

I'd taken the Monday after the disastrous Oscars off to wallow at
home. But I went right back to work the next day. It was Grandma
Ruby's voice propelling me forward. I was suddenly five years old again
and she was telling me not to let anyone push me around. That if I quit,
if I walked away from this dream, I'd be exactly what I feared the most.
I thought back on my time in college and how the administration was
intent on kicking me out. I'd learned then that you can't let people take
opportunities away from you, and it almost happened again. I'd been
working toward this moment with Rachel for years. I'd seen people get
close to their dream. But that's usually when the work gets hardest
and they throw up their hands and walk away, just before the
finish line. They say, "What I have is good enough." But you can do
more. *I* can do more. I developed a tougher skin. I insisted Taylor open the lines of communication and
keep me informed. I stood up for myself, and it made all the difference.
And soon we were working hand in hand, supporting each other.

> "Reality TV was a magnifying glass, I was finding out; by being myself, I'd given others the courage to do the same."

I don't regret crying on TV. It was such a real moment. But somehow
people saw it as a weakness. And it was hard to escape. I took solace in the
fan mail, however. Young gay kids across the country were reaching out
to me, telling me how I'd given them hope. I'd given them the courage to
come out, or to pursue their fashion dreams, or even to wear a shrunken
blazer to school. Reality TV was a magnifying glass, I was finding out; by
being myself, I'd given others the courage to do the same.

Life was moving quickly. I was making contacts, befriending fashion
publicists, and getting better at my job. I could get a look pulled from
another shoot and sent to Rachel's studio. When a client was on tour

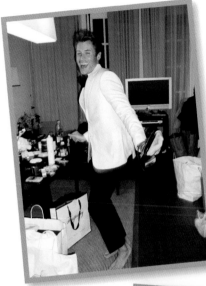

For the premiere party for the first season of *The Rachel Zoe Project*, I wanted to do a Clark Gable/*Casablanca* thing. I only had an hour to get ready. But when I saw that the pieces were working, I did a little dance.

I hung out with Nate Berkus and Andy Cohen at the premiere party. It was so hot inside my glasses were fogging up. We'd finished filming months ago. But this was the first night that it all felt real.

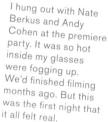

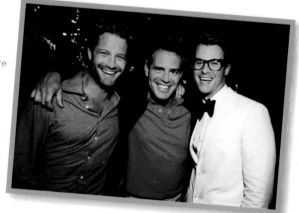

overseas and wanted to see new options at her hotel, I made the clothing appear. It was a two-way street, and the publicists knew they could trust me. If they needed a dress back from me quickly, as long as a client didn't need it, I produced it.

The job was not without challenges. There were times when I was overseas, calling Rachel at all hours of the night, texting her images of

Big Girls Don't Cry

OR HOW TO CRY LIKE A MAN, IN THREE EASY STEPS!

1. When you feel the tears coming on, try as hard as possible to stuff them back down. That's the first step. I can't control it. It's like someone with irritable bowel syndrome. Except it's tears coming down my cheeks instead of, well, you know.

2. If the tears do start coming, let them fall as if you're Demi Moore in *Ghost* and Patrick Swayze is behind you, and you can feel his presence. Those are perfect tears. If you don't know what I'm talking about, go back and rewatch the movie. You weren't watching close enough the first time.

3. If steps 1 and 2 fail, let her rip. Allow yourself to have a full-on meltdown cry to the point that you think people should be concerned for you. For the first part, look as ugly as you want to. Then bring it back in and make it a cute cry. No one wants to console an ugly crier.

dresses. Times when I wasn't sleeping. When I was up all night trying to make new outfits appear out of thin air. I was flying on private planes and having dinners in secluded rooms at five-star restaurants in exotic cities, dealing with problems that came up around the world. It was not unusual for someone to love a dress in the fitting and then want new options on the day of her event.

Was this a dream come true? In so many ways, yes. My phone would ring and I'd find myself telling friends that I was in Paris

> "I was flying on private planes and having dinners in secluded rooms at five-star restaurants in exotic cities."

shopping for Cameron Diaz. We started working together around the film
What Happens in Vegas. Before the Japanese press tour for that film, I
took a vacation with her family, traveling through Japan, doing a one-
week tour of Kyoto, Hakone, and Tokyo. I found myself in situations I
would only have dreamed of a year before. I was changing Kate Hudson

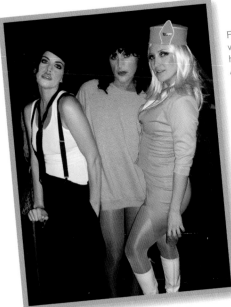

For Halloween 2008, I
went to Kate Hudson's
house party in Los
Angeles. I dressed
as Jennifer Beals in
Flashdance. Liv Tyler
(left) was a sexy Charlie
Chaplin. And our hostess
was a Pan Am stewardess.

In February of 2009, I went to
Milan for Fashion Week. This
was backstage at my first Louis
Vuitton show. I'd been saving this
three-piece Yves Saint Laurent
suit for a special occasion, and
this felt right. As for the ears,
that season there was a punk/
mid-eighties/French boudoir
inspiration to the Louis Vuitton
show. Backstage, I had to try on
the twisted bunny ears. A few
months later, Madonna wore
these same ears to the Met Ball.

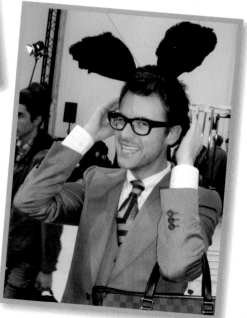

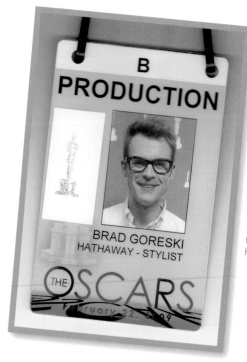

B
PRODUCTION

BRAD GORESKI
HATHAWAY - STYLIST

THE OSCARS
February 22, 2009

I was backstage at the Oscars on February 22, 2009. You forget what a clusterfuck it can be with limousines and parking. I actually thought we were going to be late. The badge helped.

out of her green Galliano into a Balmain minidress in the bathroom of Nobu before going to a party on the Thames. It's not just the glamour or the celebrity that thrilled me. Rather, we were this traveling band of gypsies—with the star and the hair-and-makeup team and the publicist and the photographers. For a moment in time, a specific but excellent moment, you became a family. And when you came back to L.A., you all went your separate ways. But when the family reunited for the next tour, you picked up right where you left off.

Between fashion shoots and awards seasons, there were surreal moments, too. Like when Mattel invited Rachel to the Barbie factory and presented her with a Barbie made in her likeness. I assumed Barbie would come from heaven. But actually, she lived in Inglewood, near LAX. My

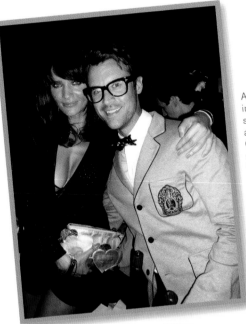

At the Marc Jacobs show in September 2009, I sat next to Kim Gordon and across from Helena Christensen. I could barely speak. As for this jacket, I bought it in Japan. The Thom Browne cut is a big thing in Japan. They have baby clothes everywhere.

Mert and Marcus shot Scarlett Johansson for a Moët campaign, and Rachel was the stylist. This was taken on the roof of the Château Marmont after the shoot.

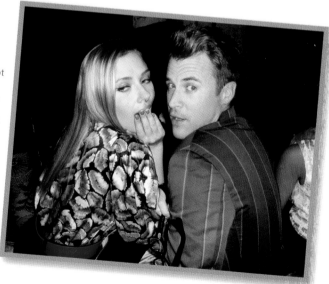

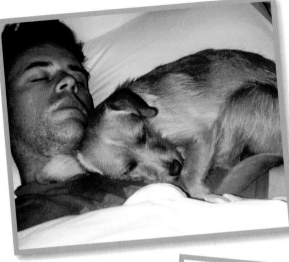

In November 2009, Gary and I adopted Penelope—a rescue dog. This was the second night we had her, and she slept on my shoulder. She still does. I keep this photo on my phone, and any time things get crazy, I look at this photo and it reminds me of what is important in life.

I met Donatella Versace for the first time in February 2010, backstage at her show in Milan. I'm wearing a Dsquared² blazer—the D, in this case, stands for Donatella. She's holding a red marabou coat. She did not disappoint. She never does. For the rest of my life, I will have butterflies around her.

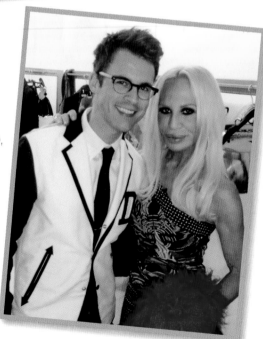

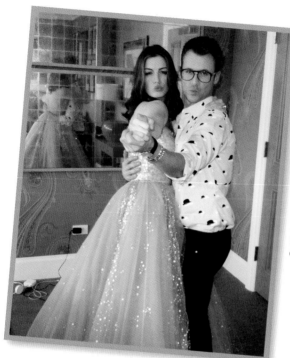

Anne Hathaway wore a gorgeous Valentino dress to the 2010 Met Ball. But the dress had been reconstructed. At the fitting, we had to make sure Anne could move around in it. I was happy to dance with her.

mind was blown. We were in the actual workshop, and there were different Barbie heads all around and endless hair options. The shelves were full of every Barbie you can imagine: *Wizard of Oz* Barbie, Marilyn Monroe Barbie, Barbie dressed in Bob Mackie. But what freaked me out the most were the shoes. When I was a kid playing with Barbie in the basement, I would always lose one of her shoes. And who wants to play with her once she loses a shoe? But here at the factory, they had bins and bins full of single shoes. What's more, everyone who worked there talked about Barbie as if she was a real person. No one referred to her as a doll. They said things like, "Barbie likes to wear her makeup like this." Or "Barbie loves her closet." I aspire to speak like this. At the factory, I told a story from my childhood. My grandmother Ruby had given me a set of Barbie

It's Barbie's World. We Just Live in It.

WHAT YOU CAN LEARN FROM BARBIE

1. The art of dressing up. It's possible to look fabulous in any scenario. Whether you're an astronaut, a teacher, a scientist, or in Malibu.
2. That nothing matters as long as you drive a pink convertible.
3. That imagination is everything. Barbie is built perfectly, but she's not really about being thin. She's about endless possibilities and dreaming big. She will be whatever you want her to be. As long as that includes being beautiful and glamorous.

dolls called Barbie and the Rockers. This was when Barbie started a girl band, and I set up their stage in our family living room. I loved those dolls, but when I came home from school, they were gone. My father had thrown the whole thing in the garbage, and I wasn't to ask any questions.

"I don't think you make Barbie and the Rockers anymore," I said at the factory. "I tried to buy it on eBay." When I finished telling this story, a press rep disappeared down a hallway and emerged with a brand-new set of Barbie and the Rockers, still in the box. It sits on the shelf in my office now, and every time I look at it I smile.

I got sick on a Lancôme commercial with Anne Hathaway, and I quit smoking cold turkey. I was up all night with a fever, I didn't have a cigarette for a week, and that was it. Giveth and taketh away. It wasn't easy. I had night sweats. I was moody and agitated. I ate more—a lot more. Let me tell you: It was harder to quit cigarettes than to give up anything else. I should mention, being sober and in fashion is a challenge. But it's not like it's 1964 and I'm the only one clean in the room. There are lots of people in fashion who don't drink. It's been ten years, and there are days where I wish I could check out. But I don't kid myself. None of this would be possible if I had a cocktail.

The ratings for the second season of *The Rachel Zoe Project* were on the rise, and the third season would be even bigger. Though it would come with changes. Shortly before we started taping, Taylor was fired. I was devastated. The first six weeks on the job might have been a horror show, but Taylor and I had developed a genuinely healthy working relationship. We'd do pulls for each other. Even though we sat across from each other all day, when we'd get our cell phone bills at the end of the month we'd laugh at how much time we'd spent talking out of the office. Our jobs were less compartmentalized, and we were more of a team. Out of loyalty to Rachel, I did not keep in touch with Taylor. But I did learn so much from her.

In life, one day we will all work for someone like Taylor—someone with that kind of strong personality. You'll probably be afraid of him or her and you'll worry that you'll never be able to please them. But these are sometimes the best teachers. From Taylor, I learned to keep it moving. She'd say those words on set all the time, "Keep it moving." An hour before a shoot wrapped, we'd be packed up and ready to messenger

> **"I don't want to say Taylor taught me to be a man, but she taught me to assert myself. And for that I will be forever grateful."**

clothing back to the designers. Under Taylor, everything flowed smoothly. I also learned to fight back. That doesn't mean you need to have your fists up, but you can't let people walk all over you, either. And sometimes, you need to give people time to let their deeper selves show through. Taylor and I didn't get along at the outset, but we grew to be close friends. Give people time and you will see beyond the exterior. When I was traveling and the shit sometimes hit the fan, Taylor was up at three in the morning with her phone in her hand, sending e-mails on my behalf. In a way, she made me less afraid—in front of clients, in front of celebrities. It's funny, in a weird way she taught me everything Dr. Zucker was supposed to teach me. I don't want to say Taylor taught me to be a man, but she taught me to assert myself. And for that I will be forever grateful.

She also taught me when it was time to leave a job. It was no mystery to anyone in town that Taylor was unhappy. She said it on TV before every commercial break. I thought she was all talk. I thought she'd work for Rachel forever. But I was wrong. She was overseeing Rachel's business, and I think she liked the power and the association that came with it. And I think she was too afraid to make the leap. Too afraid to say her time was up and she was tired of her job. Maybe in the end she was looking for a way out. She needed a push, and she got it. When I decided to leave Rachel, it was because I wanted to leave before that point came. I wanted to leave while it was all still magical. Because it was.

It was the third season and I was suddenly thrust into a leading role, cast as Rachel's style director, and every job came to me. It was a huge opportunity and overwhelmingly stressful. We styled Demi for the cover of *Harper's Bazaar.* We styled Cameron, Kate, and Eva for the Golden Globes. I fit Ashton Kutcher for his trip to Russia with Demi—which got canceled. We went to New York for Fashion Week and styled the Relief for Haiti show for Naomi Campbell. Rachel had Naomi coming down hard on her, which led to friction between us. There was a blizzard and I was expected to have clothing donated for free, two days before the show.

> **"This is what it feels like to be alive. I can see how much I've matured. And how much Rachel respects me."**

Still, not only was it an honor to work this event but I also felt like I was in the documentary *Unzipped,* the one about Isaac Mizrahi that I watched at the video store where I worked in high school. Except now it was me doing fittings, it was me backstage. David LaChapelle, Naomi, Chris Brown—it was a revolving door of famous faces. Naomi kept asking

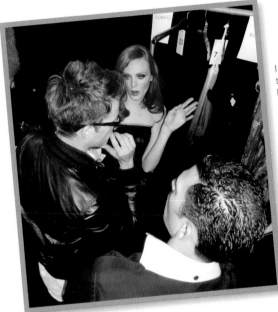

I am backstage at the Naomi Campbell benefit for Haiti during Fashion Week, consulting with Karen Elson on her look. Side note: Someone stole my green Dsquared^2 bomber jacket that day. I was so annoyed, but I put on this Bally leather jacket to console myself.

for me. "Where's Brad? Where's Brad?" In a good way! Karen Elson, Natasha Poly, and Sasha Pivovarova—these huge models—were worried they were in the wrong looks. And I was helping them to get dressed. And at the same time, despite all the chaos, the thought going through my head was a simple but essential one: I'm alive. This is what it feels like to be alive. I can see how much I've matured. And how much Rachel respects me. She and I are working this event like a team. I'm not some B-assistant trying to prove myself. We were offering up accessories, saying to each other, "What do you think of this? Should I add this in?" It was a major turning point.

People were noticing me. And I started to feel differently about myself. I started to feel stronger. It was April 2010, and we were shooting Cameron Diaz for the cover of *Harper's Bazaar*. We were on location at the top of the Met Life building. Terry Richardson was the photographer, and we barely interacted. He and Rachel are close, so I hung back, steaming garments, making sure the clothing was organized and ready to go. Which made what happened next all the more surprising. After lunch, Terry pulled me aside and said, "I want to take your picture tomorrow."

"Uh, OK," I said. "Sure."

I didn't think he was serious. But that night, I called Danielle and Annabet to tell them what Terry said. Both of them shouted the same thing: "He's going to try to get you to take your clothes off." I got it. Terry has a reputation for getting models and actors and actresses undressed for his photos. But I brushed it off. He probably wouldn't even remember. He was probably just being polite.

Well, sure enough, the next day Terry asked to take some photos with me and Rachel. We were at Milk Studios on Sixteenth Street in New York, and the three of us were posing together. He took a few of Rachel solo. And then he asked one of his assistants to bring over his special flash camera and asked if I'd take some photos by myself. I was nervous but then I thought, Fuck it. When is Terry Richardson going to ask to take my picture again?

Of course Danielle and Annabet were right. I was posing against a white backdrop wearing a pair of cut-off denim Levi's shorts I made myself; a cashmere red, white, and blue Band of Outsiders T-shirt; red Band of Outsiders suspenders; and Converse sneakers. Basically, I was dressed for kindergarten. And Terry asked me to flex my arm.

"You have a really nice biceps," he said. "What's your body like underneath your shirt? Take your shirt off."

I hesitated but then did it.

"You have abs, man!" Terry said. "Who would have known?"

Soon enough, everyone would know. A month went by and I'd almost forgotten about the photos. Until I got a tweet from someone saying, "OMG. Photos of @MrBradGoreski by Terry Richardson. Amazing."

I clicked, and I was beyond nervous. When the photos came up, I had two reactions. One: That can't be me. And two: I'm elated. Terry caught me at the right moment. I felt like Nicole Kidman in *Moulin Rouge.* She'd never looked better. And I thought I'd never look as good as I did in those photos.

The pictures were all over the Internet—me, without a shirt on. I called Gary to give him a heads-up. But it was too late. Within an hour, every fashion blog was linking to the photos. Terry later told me that it was the second-most trafficked photo on his site—after only Mary-Kate Olsen. I guess there was a desire to see me without my shirt on.

This is one of those moments in life where I'm so glad I didn't say no. Like going to Greece. Or moving to Los Angeles to be with Gary, or going to work for Rachel. I took a chance. It was a risk. And it paid off. I'd long since lost the weight from my childhood fat days, but on the inside, I still felt like the kid from Port Perry who wore a T-shirt in the pool until he was eighteen years old. My bow ties and glasses had almost become a caricature; they were as much my shield as my grunge look was in high school. I don't think people even knew I had a body under there. But I'd been working out every morning, and the gym was as much about vanity as it was about having a meditative experience. About doing something for myself, because I was worth it.

> "I took a chance. It was a risk. And it paid off."

When Terry asked to take my picture, I thought, Don't be the fat kid running away again. Just let go. And I'm so glad I did.

Working for Rachel was the best professional experience of my life. I left, in part, because I didn't want to be another Taylor. I didn't want to leave so abruptly. I didn't want to tape another season of the show and be miserable on air. I didn't want to take being on set for granted. I remembered how I felt hustling for that Kate Hudson job on my first trip to London for Rachel. It wasn't that my work was slipping, but I didn't feel that drive in my heart anymore. In the dance world, there's this phrase: "You have to eat nails." That's how badly you need to want it. And I didn't want it like that anymore. The fire was out. The only way to get that back was to work for myself.

It was time for some fresh blood to come into Rachel's studio. I didn't want to be looking for an agent behind her back. I didn't want to be setting up other jobs. I wanted to be up-front with her. I wanted her to know why I was leaving. The thought came on quickly, and the feeling in my heart was contentment. But while I was busier than I'd ever been, I was also on autopilot. And there was this nagging question at the back of my throat: Is it enough? Looking back, at every point in my life I've always thought, What is next? I was a good assistant. But if you're not making mistakes, you're not growing. Could I do more? Should I do more? Was it time to take a chance?

> "When Terry asked to take my picture, I thought, Don't be the fat kid running away again. Just let go. And I'm so glad I did."

By the time I went out on tour with Cameron Diaz for *Knight and Day,* a movie where Tom Cruise was an international spy and Cameron repaired automobiles (don't ask questions), I'd already made up my mind to leave. The press tour took me to Brazil, Mexico City, London, Salzburg, Munich, New York, and Chicago. We were in Seville, Spain, when it hit me: I could do this on my own. I was in a foreign country about to travel to another international city. I knew how to get dresses sent to me in Europe. When I took a job, the talent was happy. The publicist was happy. The studio was happy. It wasn't just that I felt secure in my duties. I used to rely on Rachel, e-mailing her photos of a client, wondering if I'd gotten it right or asking for help with securing

> "The fire was out. The only way to get that back was to work for myself."

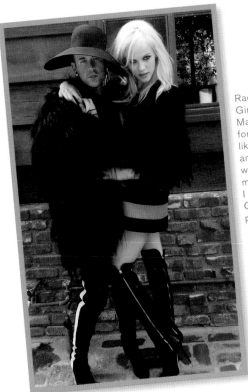

Rachel styled the model Ginta for *Love* magazine in May 2010. It was a rough day for me, as I'd decided I was likely going to leave Rachel and that this special time was coming to an end. To make the day more bearable, I dressed up and surprised Ginta. I asked her who was prettier, and she said me.

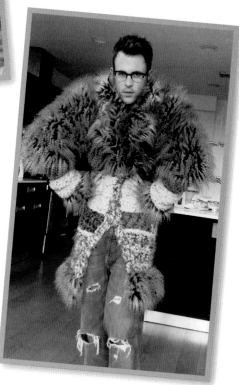

This is me in a Chanel coat. I have a habit of trying on the clothing before we shoot. Can you blame me?

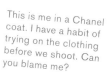

additional looks at the last minute. Rachel had been the best guide. But now she felt more like a safety net.

The truth is, others saw it first. It was other people who saw that it was time for me to move on. They knew it before I believed it in my bones. While on the *Knight and Day* tour, I hit it off with the makeup artist Gucci Westman, who does Cameron's makeup. Gucci Westman is major. She

> "But if you're not making mistakes, you're not growing."

had her big break in 1996, covering bikers in mud for an Annie Leibovitz shoot for *Vanity Fair*. Later she was named the artistic director for Lancôme. She works with Cameron and Julianne Moore and a handful of other A-list actresses. And in Rio, she told me that *Harper's Bazaar* was going to do a feature on her, celebrating her personal style. The magazine asked her for a list of people to style the shoot, and she'd submitted my name. Somehow, the magazine agreed and Rachel signed off on the job.

Back in New York, I was pulling clothing for Gucci Westman, styling a *Harper's* shoot on my own. She has serious fashion in her blood. Her husband is one of the men behind Rag & Bone. Her opinion matters. Her style is very New York, downtown cool with a European edge. She likes distressed jeans and Lanvin and vintage Cartier. Her look is disheveled chic. I called in pieces from Chanel, Dries Van Noten, and Hermès. I'd grown into my own entity. And people were starting to ask me when I was going to strike out on my own. At first, I was taken aback. But then I realized: It is time. When you no longer need a safety net, that's when it's time to take a leap.

When things are right, I believe the pieces all fall together naturally. As confusing as the universe can be, when the sign comes the pieces are usually already in place. It was time to listen to my own voice again. Comfort can be your worst enemy. Mistakes are essential to growing—whether it's a sartorial mistake or one that leads to a failed relationship.

These are the building blocks of who we are. If everything is going smoothly you're not challenging yourself. But how to do it? Again, I went to the people I admired most to ask for advice.

Prabal Gurung is a rising star in the design world, and we've come to be close friends. He graduated from Parsons School of Design—where Donna Karan, Marc Jacobs, and Jack and Lazaro from Proenza Schouler all studied—and he spent two years working with Cynthia Rowley before becoming the design director at Bill Blass. In February of 2009 he launched his own collection. I was sent photos of a few pieces before the presentation and I was blown away. I thought the clothes were stunning. They were exquisitely made—and so luxurious. The use of feathers and color made my head spin. We *needed* these clothes for Rachel's girls. Right after the presentation I attacked his PR director, Caitlin, and requested two dresses for Demi Moore—both of which she'd wear to events. The first was a black-and-white asymmetrical dress, which she wore to a Cartier party. Shortly thereafter, we dressed Demi in a Prabal Gurung

> "People were starting to ask me when I was going to strike out on my own. At first, I was taken aback. But then I realized: It is time."

asymmetrical dress with a feathered ombré skirt for the launch of the perfume Wanted, which she was the face of. Demi tweeted a photo of herself in that dress, saying, "Wonderful young designer to look out for, Prabal Gurung!" And his business exploded. Michelle Obama wore a red, matte jersey, hand-stitched draped dress by Prabal Gurung to the White House Correspondents' Dinner in May 2010. And in November 2010, Prabal was the runner-up for the Vogue/CFDA prize, awarded by Anna Wintour herself.

And so I wanted to pick his brain. Prabal and I had dinner at Bond Street. He'd successfully built his brand, leaving the comfort—and high-profile perch—he had at Bill Blass to run his own outfit. I'd seen him grow his business from nothing. I wanted to know: How did he do it? What advice could he offer me?

"There are a lot of people warming up around the teat," he said. "It's very easy to get carried away with people saying how fabulous you are. Our industry is full of that. Make sure the end goal is clear. There will be people who love you and equally people who are going to hate you. You just have to keep your head firmly on your shoulders."

As we ate lots of sushi and sashimi, Prabal said, "Talent and charm can only take you so far. Humility is the utmost key for success. All the hype and the attention is very short-lived. You should be interested in longevity." When the night was over, he said, "This is not the beginning of Brad the Fabulous. It's the beginning of Brad the Stylist. You have to pound the pavement."

He was right. I wasn't leaving Rachel because she changed. I was leaving because I changed. Because I had something to say.

It's painful when the universe sends you that moment of clarity, when the universe suggests you shake things up. Especially when that message comes during a tough job market and a worse economy. You wonder: Will I ever get work again? Is this a rash decision? Am I throwing away a good opportunity? And those were just the questions Gary asked me. I had my own concerns. But the fear felt good. It felt *right*. I just needed to trust myself and do it.

> "Humility is the utmost key for success."

It was early summer 2010 and I was staying at the Trump SoHo with Rachel. We were in town for an event, and Danielle Nachmani—my friend from the *Vogue* internship—came by the hotel for dinner. She was working for Annabel Tolman, a celebrity stylist who had been the fashion director at *Interview* magazine and is known for styling celebrities like Scarlett Johansson and America Ferrera with a rock and roll, but still feminine, sensibility. Danielle had decided she was going to leave and work with clients on her own.

"I'm leaving Annabel," Danielle said.

I was impressed and emboldened. Danielle was signed by an agency, Starworks Artists, she explained, and she was branching out on her own. As she filled me in on her news, the two of us leaned in close. It was a huge moment.

Rachel hadn't planned to join us for dinner, but she popped into the restaurant to say hello. She sat down at the table for a drink, and after Danielle broke her news, Rachel began to give her advice on starting

> "This is not the beginning of Brad the Fabulous. It's the beginning of Brad the Stylist."

her business. Later, Rachel would say this was the night she knew she'd lost me. The moment she walked into the restaurant and saw Danielle and I huddled together, she knew I'd be leaving soon.

When I finally made the move, I was terrified. I was calling Rachel, and she was putting it off. Because she knew. Finally, I sent her a text that said, "I really need to talk to you today." Because I knew if I didn't do it right then, I was going to chicken out.

When I sat down with Rachel and Rodger, I was very explicit about the reasons why I wanted to leave. That I wanted to try and see what styling on my own would be like. I gave Rachel more than two months' notice and stayed past my end date to finish out a photo shoot with her. I was very honest with them—that I had this strong feeling inside of myself that it was time for us to part ways. But I was adamant about the fact that

I didn't want this to prevent us from being friends and it was my hope that when I left we'd be able to continue to talk on the phone and text and do all of the things that we used to do. Although this has been questioned, I

> "The fear felt good. It felt *right*."

have never solicited a client of hers. I will always credit her with being a great teacher and boss and I'm so grateful to have had the opportunity to work with her. I was ready to go out on my own. And yet in so many ways, I wasn't ready at all. Was I making a leap? Or jumping into the abyss?

LEAP

9

Take risks and be bold.
And not just in fashion.

THOUGH I WOULDN'T ANNOUNCE my split from
Rachel Zoe until September 29, I'd actually given her my
notice in July. We agreed to keep the news quiet until after
New York Fashion Week. And now here it was. While it
was liberating to make my own Fashion Week schedule, I
was also freaking out. People were inviting me to parties
and to shows. But why? I was a TV personality without a
TV show. I was a stylist without any clients.

The week was nonstop. The *New York Times* sent a
reporter to follow me around to write a profile of me as
the "breakout star" of *The Rachel Zoe Project*. (I struggled
not to tell the writer that I'd already left the show.) I was

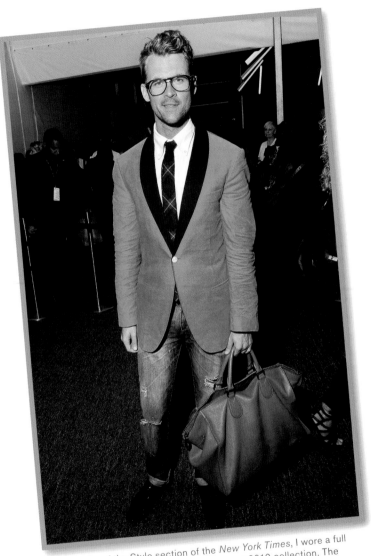

For the cover of the Style section of the *New York Times*, I wore a full Michael Bastian look from his Spring/Summer 2010 collection. The bag is Louis Vuitton, and this is one of my favorite runway looks. Color always looks good in photographs. I wore this because it fit perfectly and didn't need alterations, and because I knew I'd never regret it.

interviewed by TV crews, giving my reactions to the collections. I sat front row at Simon Spurr's presentation, alongside Matt Bomer from *White Collar* (hot). His was a full runway show, and Simon's clothes were the definition of exquisite British tailoring, with three-piece suits and waistcoats, in a palette grounded in neutrals with yellow, pink, and

> "I was a TV personality without a TV show. I was a stylist without any clients."

blue woven into it. I was interviewed by TV crews for my reactions to the collections. I sat front row at Alexander Wang.

Before the Alexander Wang show, I met up with Rachel, Rodger, and Rachel's sister Pam. We had lunch outside Pastis, and the moment felt celebratory and sad all at once. I'd made Rachel a photo album of pictures of the two of us from the past two years and eight months together—photos from Paris Fashion Week, photos from the first season premiere

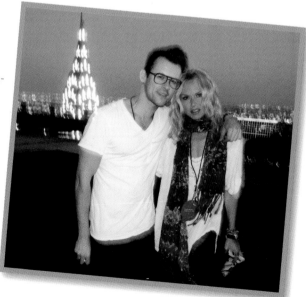

Terry Richardson shot Cameron Diaz for the cover of *Harper's Bazaar*. We shot all day on this roof, with Cameron standing around in this gold, long-sleeved Balmain dress while Terry was blasting Alicia Keys and Jay-Z's "Empire State of Mind." Rachel and I posed for this photo during an amazing moment as we watched the city lights come on.

party for the TV show, photos of us with Terry Richardson. We flipped through the album together at the restaurant and we both began to cry, big heaving sobs. It was heartbreaking. I knew it was the end of a very special era and a time that I would never have again. I wished that our relationship would continue. We'd shared this wild experience together that was *The Rachel Zoe Project.* But I felt like this was a good-bye. And there was so much sadness.

> "It was heartbreaking. I knew it was the end of a very special era and a time that I would never have again."

I formally announced my split from Rachel in September 2010 in the pages of *People* magazine, saying, in a prepared statement, "There's a point where either I do it now or I'll never know what it's like to spread my wings and soar."

Yet why did I feel like my wings had been clipped?

The work wasn't just slow, it was nonexistent. And when it did come, it was comical in only the way things in my life can be. I was still the outsider looking in. My first job on my own was for *Entertainment Weekly,* styling Anne Hathaway and Jake Gyllenhaal for the cover, timed to the release of their Oscar hopeful, *Love and Other Drugs.* The magazine had offered the gig to Rachel, but she was pregnant and unavailable to fly to New York. When they called

> "I loved that. I worked for one of the best stylists in the world, but I needed my best friend to tell me to edit."

me, believe me, I was on the next flight out. I flew myself to New York and would lose money on the job, but I was desperate to keep my name out there. There was some speculation that I wanted to poach Anne Hathaway. If anything, I would have poached Jake, who works with the stylists Nina and Clare Hallworth—a.k.a. the Twins. I wanted to establish myself as a men's stylist, and he was on my list of dream clients.

I came to New York for the first time as a small-business owner. And it was a different world. This time, I wasn't staying at the Mercer or the Crosby. I was crashing with my friend Annabet, whom I'd met the first summer I spent in New York. It was a reality check. It was also the best slumber party in the world and a learning experience. I had called in clothing from every major men's designer for the *EW* job. Messengers were showing up to Annabet's apartment at all hours. I had every boot. I had every shoe. She came home one night to find a dozen racks in her living room. She looked around the apartment and laughed, "Babe, you need to learn how to edit."

> **"I felt like the fat kid in my childhood bedroom all over again, staring up at the stars and wondering what was next for me."**

I loved that. I worked for one of the best stylists in the world, but I needed my best friend to tell me to edit.

In the end, the joke was on me. I got to the shoot. I was setting up the racks, opening boxes and laying accessories out on a table. I had so much clothing I actually stopped opening boxes because there was no room. Meanwhile, Jake and Anne were so comfortable with each other that they decided to pose naked, with Jake's gorgeous ripped arm draped around Anne. I got a styling credit, but there was no clothing in the photo. It was my first cover and there were two credits: a pair of boxer shorts and a bra.

I felt like the fat kid in my childhood bedroom all over again, staring up at the stars and wondering what was next for me. Wondering how I could make this happen. More than ever, I wanted to call my grandma Ruby for advice. Whenever something big happens in my life I want to call her. At least, I was excited again. I could feel the promise in my bones, the anticipation. In a way, I flashed back to how I felt during my very first New York Fashion Week, after my internship at *Vogue*. I was about to start my sophomore year in college, and Annabet was an associate fashion editor at *Jane* magazine. She'd taken a freelance gig for Fashion Week, styling a runway show for the Los Angeles–based jewelry designer Chris Aire. The show was major. There were twenty-five million dollars' worth of diamonds on display. Wyclef Jean performed. Tyson Beckford walked. Isabeli walked. (Fun fact: This was Rosie Huntington-Whiteley's first-ever runway show.) In the days leading up to the event, Annabet was so overwhelmed with fittings and stylings that she couldn't attend any other runway shows. So she called me: "Come by the hotel and you can have all of my tickets. Everything is RSVP'd for already." And I did, playing pretend that year, walking into those shows acting as if I belonged.

> "Now here I was again, fighting to prove myself, playing dress-up and pretending."

Now here I was again, fighting to prove myself, playing dress-up and pretending. I was back to New York often that fall for an endless stream of meetings. I was banging the drum, trying to build up business. And I was crashing with Annabet in her twenty-ninth-floor one-bedroom in the financial district. Her apartment was largely empty, which felt like a metaphor for something. I had Annabet's keys. Her doorman knew me by face and by name. Annabet was going through a breakup, and in a way, so was I. We could have been miserable. But not everything had to be so serious. Instead, we decided to go out and enjoy the best city in the world. Who knew when we'd have this time again? And so, it was a lot of late nights of dancing and mayhem. We played "Hot Tottie" by Usher and Jay-Z. We had impromptu dance parties in her apartment. We were out every night of the week. At the Chanel party. At the Proenza after-party. We went to Cafeteria in Chelsea at five in the morning, like we were twenty-two-year-old interns all over again. We fell asleep at the table eating shepherd's pie. In the morning, I actually forgot that we ate. I felt something heavy in my stomach and turned to Annabet, asking, "We ate last night?" We were like college students again, eating deep-fried Oreos. At night, we'd be all dressed up—the perfect fashion couple—and the

New York, New York

MY FAVORITE MANHATTAN RESTAURANTS

ABC Kitchen, 35 East Eighteenth Street

When I'm right off the plane, this is usually my first stop for dinner. The space is beautiful: a whitewashed room of bleached wood and this harvest table where they display the fresh ingredients. My must-have meal: carrot and avocado salad, fried chicken, and the salted caramel sundae. Delish.

Arturo's, 106 West Houston Street

I usually stay at the Mercer Hotel when I'm in New York, just down the street from Arturo's. If I'm staying in for the night, I'll order a pepperoni pizza from Arturo's and have it delivered to the room. Nothing beats it.

One Lucky Duck, 125 East Seventeenth Street

During Fashion Week, One Lucky Duck is my go-to spot for a quick health fix. It's across from Milk Studios, so it's a big fashion hangout. My recommendation: the blue-green algae smoothie.

Locanda Verde, 377 Greenwich Street

Chef Andrew Carmellini can do no wrong. Every dish here—from the lamb meatball sliders to the fennel-glazed duck—is flawless.

Il Buco, 47 Bond Street

Two words: kale salad.

Gemma, 335 Bowery

On a brisk New York morning, there's nowhere better for an outdoor breakfast. I sit at a table on the Bowery, order the baked eggs cooked in the wood-fired oven, and read *Women's Wear Daily*. It's also great for people-watching.

(CONTINUED ON NEXT PAGE)

Balthazar, 80 Spring Street
On a cold winter day, stop in for a ginger tea in the late afternoon.
Ginger is good for your health, and this cup will warm you right up.

Lupa, 170 Thompson Street
Delicious Italian. Try the chicken diavola and the ever-changing
menu of seasonal desserts.

Gramercy Tavern, 42 East Twentieth Street
A great place for dinner with your family. On the way out, the staff
will hand you a little fresh-baked muffin for breakfast, which is the
chicest touch.

doorman would ask us where we were heading. Meanwhile, we'd come
back at five in the morning trying to avoid eye contact with him, like
little kids in trouble. Because we looked like the party machine spit us
out. My hair would be flat, I'd be missing a button, and my bow tie
would be askew.

We were regulars at the Boom Boom Room, at the top of the
Standard Hotel, a glass palace of high glamour that opened on the High
Line. Halloween that year was major. I was attending a party for Lanvin,
and Annabet and I decided to dress up like our favorite fashion bloggers.
It was all very fashion-forward. I had nothing but free time, and so I
called Annabet. "Meet me at Ricky's," I demanded.

And we scoured the party store for costume embellishments. Annabet
dressed up as Jane Aldridge from Sea of Shoes, wearing Dolce & Gabbana.
I dressed up as Tavi Gevinson, the teenage blogger and muse of Karl
Lagerfeld who is flown all over the world to attend fashion shows. I wore a
purple wig and a full Louis Vuitton look and clear glasses—a look ripped
directly from her blog. At the party, people were freaking out. The next
day Tavi tweeted me saying she loved it. That night was everything. And

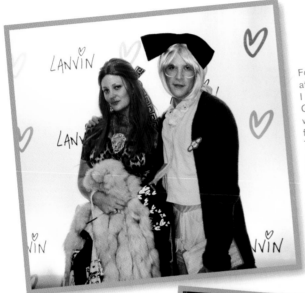

For a Halloween party at the Lanvin store, I dressed as Tavi Gevinson and Annabet went as Jane Aldridge from Sea of Shoes. There's nothing else to say about this amazing photograph.

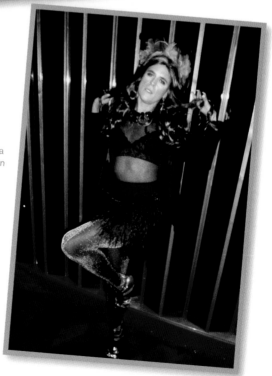

I borrowed this Louis Vuitton look from the showroom for my Anna Dello Russo Halloween costume, and I have more legs than a bucket of chicken.

Men Behaving Badly

THREE FASHION MISTAKES WE NEED TO CORRECT

1. Embroidered jeans with embellishments
Not a good look—on anyone.

2. The super-deep V-neck
If you have a great chest, there are other ways to show it off. Wear a button-down shirt and leave an extra button open. Or buy a traditional V-neck T-shirt in a tighter cut. But leave some mystery.

3. The boxy suit
Once a month, take a few pieces to the tailor. Those oversize suits? The ones with the drop shoulders and the jacket that goes down to your knees? That's not a flattering look. Breathe new life into those suits by having them taken in. Even the most inexpensive suit can look great with the right tailoring.

the next day was more of the same. There were more parties, more chances to remind people that I was out there and available. For another party, Annabet and I went to Sephora and I put on a full trans face. I dressed up as Anna Dello Russo, an editor at large for *Vogue* Japan and a fashion icon. Annabet was Brigitte Bardot in red lipstick and a leopard Dolce top. That night there was a run-in with a Dolly Parton look-alike and thousands of balloons and we got in a cab with Joe Zee and Danielle Nachmani and headed to this party underneath the Chelsea Hotel.

> "They say that when you leap, a net will appear. I had to believe it would."

Maybe it was all a distraction, but it was a beautiful distraction. I had no idea when I'd ever be able to stay up until five in the morning and sleep until three again. But I confessed my deepest fears to Annabet: Was I any good? I kept saying, "Maybe I don't have anything to say." Some advice from Prabal Gurung flashed through my head: "This is not the beginning of Brad the Fabulous. It's the beginning of Brad the Stylist. You have to pound the pavement."

> "Because I was nervous, too. I was plagued by the feeling that I was out of my depth."

They say that when you leap, a net will appear. I had to believe it would.

I was at home in Los Angeles when my phone buzzed with a text from Joe Zee, a man whose work I greatly respect. Among other unforgettable shoots, he styled my all-time favorite spread of Jennifer Lopez for *W* magazine. J. Lo is photographed so often you think, How can you make this new? But Joe totally pulled it off, in a Guy Bourdin–inspired shoot, dressing her in fishnets and a bodysuit and Louboutins with her hair blowing.

The text from Joe read: "I'm on set with Jessica Alba shooting her for the cover of *Elle*. She told me her stylist is leaving. Do you want to style her?"

Um, duh.

Apparently, Jessica Alba had the vaguest sense of who I was. She knew I worked for Rachel but hadn't heard that I was now on my own. Joe put in a good word and connected me with Jessica's publicist, who promised to set up a call for Jessica and me to speak. I was at a taping of Bravo's *Watch What Happens Live* with Andy Cohen when my phone rang: Alba. I ducked out for an hour and she and I talked. She asked about my aesthetic, about the designers I like. She'd been working with her stylist for ten years, she explained, and she was concerned about finding the right person to take his place. They had a well-established relationship, and their work together had been widely applauded. Jessica Alba is known for being modern and cool but not trend-specific. She'll wear the dress of the season, but in her own way.

There was a time crunch here. The task at hand: Jessica had a press tour coming up for *Little Fockers,* with stops at the major talk shows on both coasts plus a Manhattan premiere. It would be the dead of winter on the East Coast, which presented its own challenge. The weather was only one hurdle. This was a big movie for Jessica. She was the youngest woman in the cast, and she was new to the *Fockers* franchise—suddenly thrown into the deep end of a major studio comedy alongside the likes of Ben Stiller, Robert De Niro, Blythe Danner, Dustin Hoffman, and Barbra Streisand. I appreciated her candor. Because I was nervous, too. I was plagued by the feeling that I was out of my depth. Perhaps she and I would confront this challenge together.

Before we hung up the phone, she asked me to send her a few inspiration images. She was wrapping up the fourth *Spy Kids* movie down in Austin, Texas, and we'd set up a face-to-face meeting for when she returned to L.A. The next day, I sent her three stories that inspired me. There was a big nineties Calvin Klein minimalism resurgence happening in fashion, which I loved. Prada, meanwhile, was doing a very ladylike collection at the time. I gave Jessica a cross-section of ideas that fit into different elements of her personality. And somehow, she was on board. I had no regular clients. And yet now I had a chance to land an A-list actress. This business is nothing if not fickle.

To say I had a lot riding on this fitting with Jessica Alba is the understatement of the year. Her previous stylist had tipped me off, telling me what to expect. Jessica is a mom first and foremost, he said, and she's busy. She likes clothing but only to a point. Don't show up with ten racks of clothing. Show up with one tightly edited rack. I thought, This cannot be another Anne Hathaway/Jake Gyllenhaal situation. I heard Annabet in my head saying, "Babe, you need to learn how to edit." I had to know what I wanted her to wear. She is the rare actress who doesn't like a fitting, who doesn't care about the attention. She doesn't want to spend five hours trying on dresses. When she says she'd rather be with her family, she's telling the truth.

"How will I know when the fitting is over?" I asked.

"When she sits down," he said. "That's your cue to leave." Gulp.

I pulled up to Jessica's house and her assistant let me in. I set up in the guest room, up a flight of stairs. And I was happy that I'd edited the racks—because it was like Barry's Bootcamp carrying these garment bags up that curved staircase. It was like an obstacle course. I was scared that I was going to scratch the walls with the garment bags. This was not a good way to start a fitting. Meanwhile, I set up the rack and hung up a strapless couture Valentino, white with tiers of feathers. The premiere would be held shortly before Christmas, and there was a Winter Wonderland theme happening. I had everything from Narciso Rodriguez to Prada, from Prabal Gurung to Opening Ceremony. It was a mix of fresh designers and legendary glamour. Jessica, I was finding out, doesn't care if everybody is going to love what she wears. She's not afraid of risks, and she likes what she feels

> "But these fears made me realize this was what I was supposed to be doing. I was supposed to be taking risks."

comfortable in. For a meeting she had scheduled with Revlon, we paired a bodysuit with a floral skirt for a great nineties moment. The premiere was the real challenge. She tried on the feathered Valentino but was concerned the feathers would be too cutesy. I surprised myself and pushed her, gently but firmly. You can't be a yes man, I knew. I was being paid for my point of view. I believed this dress was the strongest option, and I conveyed that. She took a second look and came around.

When word leaked out that I was working with Jessica Alba, more jobs followed. An editor at *InStyle* magazine called. They were shooting the lovely Ethiopian model Liya Kebede in a six-page story on Jil Sander's new collection and wanted me to style it. I was beside myself: This was a major national fashion magazine taking a chance on me with a big model and a huge photographer. But before I accepted the job, I asked

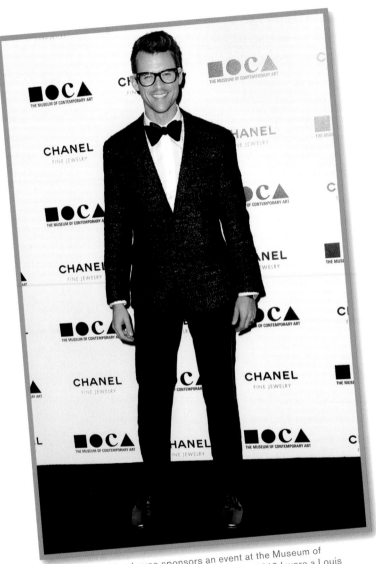

Every year a fashion house sponsors an event at the Museum of Contemporary Art in Los Angeles. In December 2010 I wore a Louis Vuitton jacket, Band of Outsiders pants, and Lanvin shoes. The jacket is gold, with this black sheared fabric. It's an updated version of men's evening wear. And it made me look very tall.

myself, What if I get to the set and people ask me questions that I can't answer? The shoot will be entirely Jil Sander looks. How can I make it look different from photographs from the runway? There were deeper questions brewing that went to the core of this transition: Could I really be an editorial stylist? But these fears made me realize this was what I was supposed to be doing. I was supposed to be taking risks.

And so I accepted the job. When I arrived on set it was more crowded than the rave clubs I used to go to in Toronto. There were two assistants, a slew of people from *InStyle,* a makeup artist and hairdresser, my agent, the photographer, his assistants, and of course a very stunning Liya Kebede. The day did not go smoothly. We needed eight looks. Unfortunately, half the clothing was held up at customs and wouldn't be arriving. Eight looks were all we had. And there was no margin for

> "Had I leaped too soon? Was this going to work out? Also: Did I have what it takes to be the boss?"

error. It was like one big puzzle. How to make it work? I was staring at the rack. What to do? *Babe, you need to learn how to edit.*

In the end, I went back to the collection. I was telling the story of this clothing, which was the reintroduction of color-blocking. Raf Simons's vision at Jil Sander was so strong, I didn't need a high concept. The clothes would speak for themselves. I needed to add the right accessories and put my touch on it. The fabrics were stiff and the cut of the clothing didn't always lend itself to movement. I thanked God we were working with a fashion model that day and not an actress. Never forget that modeling is a skill! With each look that passed, I felt a sense of relief. The shoot lasted eight hours, but it felt like an eternity. Still, I must have done something right, because the magazine later offered me a three-story contract. To have someone bet on you—and for you to deliver—is a remarkable feeling.

The phone was ringing—not steadily, but it was ringing. And my voice was developing. I'd been to a shoot in Alaska where we were calling in boots from New York—boots I was pretty sure we'd never use. Now that I was the boss, I was forcing myself to have a real reason for every item I brought. To have a strong idea as opposed to having everything there and waiting for inspiration to strike.

I was in London styling the British singer Adele for *InStyle* right after Christmas. It was a beauty shoot, which focused on the hair and makeup. For accents, I pulled jewelry from Van Cleef and Cartier and Bulgari. I pulled a sequined Dries Van Noten collared shirt dress, and some items from Michael Kors and from Mary-Kate and Ashley's line Elizabeth and James. When I arrived at the shoot, the photographer said, "Oh, I was hoping the clothing would be a little softer, a little more feminine." I'm sorry, but I wanted to say, Have you *listened* to Adele's album? The girl who sings "Rolling in the Deep" doesn't want to be wrapped in chiffon.

On my way home, I took a detour through New York and nearly missed an interview at Kate Spade thanks to a brutal snowstorm. Suddenly it was January, six months since I gave my notice. I took the temperature of my struggling business. I was busy but not busy enough. For the first time, true regret seeped in. Had I leaped too soon? Was this going to work out? Did I have what it takes to be the boss?

Demi Moore had nothing to wear. This would be a test of my skills as a stylist but also as a manager.

It was January 2011, and an e-mail from Demi Moore's manager landed in my in-box. I'd worked with Demi on and off before. She was going to Brazil and then traveling to the Sundance Film Festival in Park City, Utah, for the premiere of her film *Another Happy Day,* in which she starred opposite Ellen Barkin. A big trip, a big film, and nothing to wear.

Hey, Four Eyes!

HOW TO BUY THE RIGHT GLASSES—FOR YOU

When you're standing at the counter looking at two hundred frames, it's important to know: What is the look you're going for? Do you want something meek? Do you want a big Sally Jessy Raphael moment? (I'd die to get an actual pair of her glasses.) Do you want a big, thick nerd moment? Do you want to look like a lesbian interior designer with a rectangular clear frame?

As with anything in fashion, you're playing dress-up. You should be excited about the way you look in your glasses. Because they're going to be on your face. You should love them. Don't rush. I love Oliver Peoples—a company that has been making eyeglasses for almost thirty years. That's their business. I love Gucci and Chanel. But you don't have to spend a fortune, either. Warby Parker makes cute fashion glasses for $99 and you can buy them online.

Glasses can be a disguise. They're a barrier between you and the world. I look different in every pair I own. They give you the instant ability to take on a different look. They're an extension of who you are. The thick black nerd glasses I wore the first season of *The Rachel Zoe Project*? I chose them because I felt like a character in them. They inadvertently became part of my look. Glasses can do the same for you. So put the effort into finding the right pair.

I did a pull for Demi, spending three days shopping for Lanvin, Donna Karan, Valentino, Victoria Beckham—you name it, I had it. Plus, lots of chic high-heeled winter boots. We did a fitting in the morning, and I'd brought in a part-time assistant, Thomas Carter Phillips, to help. It was just a few hours before Demi was due at LAX, and the tailor was pinning four dresses. Everyone knew it was an extreme rush job. We arranged a pickup time for a few hours later. Double kiss, mission accomplished.

> "Suddenly it was like *The Fast and the Furious* meets *Project Runway.*"

Except that the tailor was running late and there was a miscommunication about the drop-off location. Now Demi was at the airport wondering where her dresses were. No one should be in Brazil without her best clothing. Least of all a fashion icon whom designers love and someone I was beyond desperate to land as a client.

Thomas called to break the news. He was in the car with Demi's dresses; that was the good news. But the bad news? "I have fifteen minutes to get to LAX before Demi takes off," he said.

For the first time, here I was on the other side of the coin. I was the boss. My assistant was in a rough spot. But it was my reputation on the line.

Suddenly it was like *The Fast and the Furious* meets *Project Runway.* Thomas was off and running. And I was texting him directions, telling him the best way to avoid the freeways. "Turn right on La Tijera!" I texted.

And then . . . nothing. Thomas stopped responding entirely. Has he driven off the road? I wondered. It could have happened. I mean, there were no-texting laws for a reason. Or had Thomas missed Demi's flight entirely, and now he was afraid to tell me? I couldn't decide what was worse: disappointing Demi or having Thomas die in a fiery crash.

I had two choices here. I could needle this kid and continue to call him and text him and risk alienating him. Or I could trust that he was doing everything he could to get the job done. I sympathized with him. I'd been in that position before. And I decided to leave him be. He wasn't some silly kid who thought it would be fun to work in fashion. I'd seen his work ethic on shoots. I left him alone.

But when my phone rang, I leaped for it.

"Did you get there?"

"I got the dresses to her!" Thomas said.

Fittingly, Katy Perry's "Firework" was playing in the background of the car, and it felt right. This was a cause for celebration. It was also bittersweet. I'd found a fashion assistant I respected, and I could see potential in him. But I lost him to another job, because I couldn't afford to pay him full-time.

10

Leap and the net will appear. Or you better own a pair of parachute pants.

WHEN THE *HOLLYWOOD REPORTER* released a list of the twenty-five most powerful stylists in March 2011, I was shocked to find that I was on the list. Granted, I was holding on at number twenty-two by little more than a fraying vintage thread, but there I was. The venerable trade publication wrote: "Rachel Zoe's former assistant is a rising star in the stylist world. Goreski not only landed Jessica Alba as his client (she parted ways with longtime stylist Daniel Caudill) but also got the job styling designer Kate Spade's Fall 2011 collection."

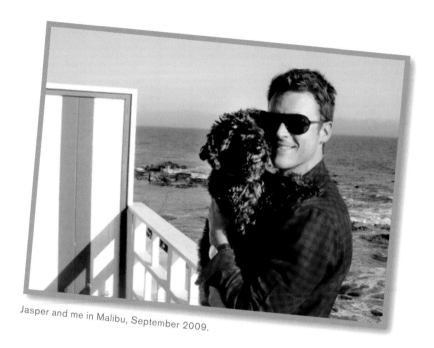

Jasper and me in Malibu, September 2009.

It's funny how something can sound so real in print when the day-to-day is still so uncertain. I had some big-name clients and a camera crew following me to shoots for a reality series called *It's a Brad, Brad World* that I was filming for Bravo. Yet, while I might have been the twenty-second-most powerful stylist in town according to the very smart, very beautiful people at the *Hollywood Reporter,* I was also still working out of my garage. UPS and FedEx men came to the house all day. Gary was writing from home some days and he was driven mad by the constant buzz of the doorbell. But I didn't have an office, and so I had no choice but to do fittings at home. When David Dean Portelli, a manager at Precision Entertainment, whom I know from Toronto, threw a job my way, asking

> "It's funny how something can sound so real in print when the day-to-day is still so uncertain."

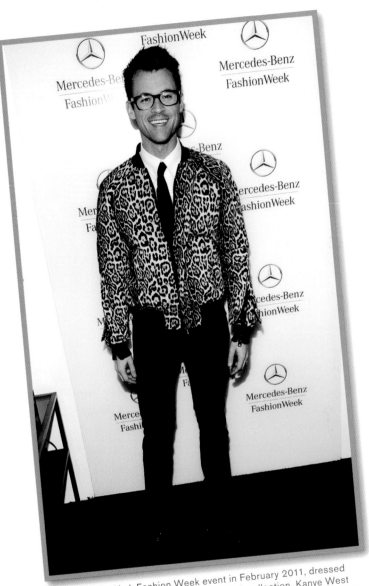

I hosted a New York Fashion Week event in February 2011, dressed in a Givenchy bomber from their spring 2010 collection. Kanye West wore this jacket right after me to Paris Fashion Week, and it turned into a major Who Wore It Better moment. I think I won.

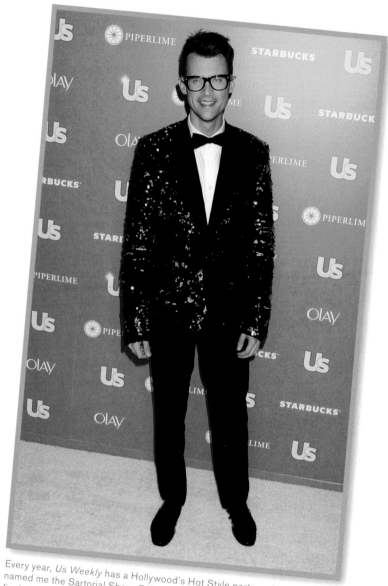

Every year, *Us Weekly* has a Hollywood's Hot Style party and in 2011 they named me the Sartorial Show-Off. And so, for the party, I showed off in a finale look from the Dolce & Gabbana Fall/Winter 2011 collection, which they shipped into Milan for me. This is my Diana Ross/Liza moment. Those sequins are everything.

if I'd like to style Shay Mitchell from *Pretty Little Liars* for the White House Correspondents' Dinner, I jumped at the chance. Shay is not only gorgeous but she's also Canadian. Yet I had to invite her over to my house for the fitting. Shay arrived late at night, coming straight from the set of *Pretty Little Liars*. Gary locked himself in the bedroom with the dogs. He wanted me to seem like a professional. Still, during the fitting, you could hear Jasper, our fifteen-year-old black miniature schnauzer,

> "He knew something I didn't yet understand: It takes money to make money."

scratching and crying on the other side of the wall. We tried gowns and cocktail dresses from J. Mendel, Jenny Packham, Phillip Lim, and Marc by Marc. The fitting didn't end until eleven thirty, and I was so exhausted I couldn't bring myself to clean up the living room. I just left the racks set up and the boxes open and splayed about. Gary wasn't angry. He was incredibly patient. But when he looked at the fashion detritus, I knew he thought I could do better.

He knew something I didn't yet understand: It takes money to make money.

It was time to take it up a notch. I hadn't been fired from a job yet.

The King of Cool

WHAT MEN CAN LEARN FROM STEVE MCQUEEN

Steve McQueen was masculine but fashionable, which isn't easy to do. It was the way he carried himself. There's that famous shot of him, carrying a cup in his hand, dressed in a turtleneck, a blazer, and a pair of pants, and he just looks so effortlessly put together, with this air of masculinity. From suits to leather jackets, he never made a mistake, and he's a constant reference for photo shoots because he walked that fine line.

Actually, my work was getting noticed and people were starting to see me as a stylist more than a TV personality. If I was still working overtime to prove myself, so be it. I had to accept that some people would see me as that guy from TV and let my work speak for itself. In some ways, I realized, I would always be that kid on the school playground, that fat kid the bullies all tormented. There will always be naysayers. But what good is it to add your own self-hating voice to that chorus? I needed to trust myself.

> "There will always be naysayers. But what good is it to add your own self-hating voice to that chorus? I needed to trust myself."

I got a call from an editor at *Details* magazine, Andrea Oliveri. The magazine wanted me to put together a few ideas for possible fashion stories. It was a great opportunity to showcase my editorial voice, and when I was out to dinner with Joe Zee later that week I ran a few thoughts by him. The ideas were good, he said, but he pushed me to pitch something more personal.

"I'm trying to stay away from bow ties and glasses," I said.

That wasn't what he meant. He told me not to be so literal and pushed me to think of something that would reflect my passion in menswear. I looked down. I was wearing a pink suit. I thought of Jil Sander's new collection, which was all about color. I was loving pops of color, I said. You can wear a bright blue shirt with a suit. There is real takeaway knowledge there.

"Pitch that!" he said. "It has to be personal."

I pitched three ideas to *Details.* That was the one they took.

I could do this. It was time to invest in myself. I was convinced: If I gave off the appearance of success, the work would follow. If I took my business seriously, others would, too. And so I needed an assistant.

I found her behind the desk at the Mercer. Or rather, she found me. For

Everything Old Is New Again

MY FIVE FAVORITE VINTAGE SHOPS—AND WHAT TO BUY THERE

1. New York Vintage, 117 West Twenty-fifth Street, New York

From Gianni Versace to Alexander McQueen, from headdresses to amazing costume jewelry, Shannon Hoey has one of the most expansive vintage collections and one of the best for vintage couture. It's a go-to spot for designers, stylists, and models.

2. Decades, 8214 Melrose Avenue, Los Angeles

Cameron Silver is not only a shop owner but also a historian and a wonderful resource for the fashion world. He specializes in vintage couture, including Valentino, Balenciaga, and Dior. Being in his store is like being in a museum. He has a fantastic collection of vintage Birkin bags and Chanel bags, and I'm always pulling from Decades for the red carpet.

3. Mint Vintage, 20 Earlham Street, London, UK

Whenever I am in London, I stop in to Mint at Seven Dials in Covent Garden to get bow ties. There is a bowl of vintage bow ties and they sell for six pounds each. Velvet, brocades, satin—it's a fantastic assortment.

4. Rose Bowl Flea Market, 1001 Rose Bowl Drive, Pasadena

On the second Sunday of every month, the crowds descend on the Rose Bowl Flea Market. It's a mixed bag, and you'll need to spend a fair amount of time sifting through. But I found a vintage navy Givenchy blazer here for $35 and a vintage Louis Vuitton trunk in perfect condition ($1,200), and it's also where I get my vintage T-shirts, sometimes ten for $10. You can't beat that.

(CONTINUED ON NEXT PAGE)

5. Didier Ludot, 20–24 Galerie Montpensier, Paris, France
This is one of the most famous vintage stores in Paris and the place where Reese Witherspoon got the Oscar gown she wore in 2006 when she won for *Walk the Line*. I bought a cream leather Christian Dior trench coat here. It's really two separate stores—one side for the general public, and then one side that's more like a museum, with mint-condition vintage Christian Dior, Balenciaga, and Balmain. But what blew me away was the sixties mod pieces—the Courrèges dresses, the patent-leather sleeves, the dress made of discs. This is the real deal.

years, whenever Gary and I traveled to New York, we stayed at the Mercer Hotel. It's very chic and timeless, and the people-watching in the lobby is a-*mahzing*. It's also a nostalgic place for me: It's the first hotel I ever stayed at in New York, when Gary took me there shortly after 9/11. Lindsay Myers had been a staple at the front desk of the Mercer for three years. She's what my grandma Ruby would have called a spark plug. Lindsay is from Hilton Head, South Carolina, and she came to New York after having a vision: She was backpacking through Fiji and Thailand after college when she saw herself surrounded by culture. On the strength of that vision, she moved to New York. I liked this girl. I liked that spirit. She was a problem solver.

I was checking out of the hotel one day before heading back to L.A., and I was complaining out loud. I had packages to pick up, and Gary was calling the front desk, wondering where I was. I was missing important conference calls. I was missing meetings because I couldn't keep my schedule straight.

"You're all over the place," Lindsay said. "You need help. You need *me*." She had no experience in fashion. She was, however, a doer. When you're the concierge at a chic Manhattan hotel, you never know what the day will bring. You're making the impossible possible every day. "What's the toughest assignment you've had?" I asked. She was discreet. But told me about a hotel guest who needed to charter a helicopter in Africa to check in on a friend in a remote village. Lindsay got that done. I thought, She can certainly handle anything I throw at her. She moved to Los Angeles on May 23. And I didn't realize how much I needed her until she was sitting next to me in my house, laughing at the disarray that was my life.

"You're a stylist," she said. "Go style. Give me the reins."

Part of me felt this was completely ridiculous. I felt like I was playing dress-up yet again—but the kind of dress-up where you don't know if your outfit is a hit or a miss. I mean, I had an assistant? I was going to look at office space? When my sister and I were little, we'd play a game in the

Hold All Calls, Miss McGill

HOW TO BE A GOOD ASSISTANT (AND IT STARTS WITH KNOWING THAT *WORKING GIRL* REFERENCE)

1. Don't add to the problem. Present solutions.
2. Honesty is the best policy.
3. Respond to every e-mail in an efficient and polite manner.
4. Try to be a step ahead. Nothing feels better than saying, "I've already taken care of that."
5. Deal with as much as possible without having your boss involved.
6. Know your boss's schedule inside and out.
7. Look the part. Be presentable every day. Even jeans and a T-shirt can look good with a little extra effort put into it.
8. Never appear tired. More important: Never say you are tired. No one cares.
9. Be early. You should be waiting for your boss, not the other way around.
10. Do everything with a smile. Or at least fake a smile.

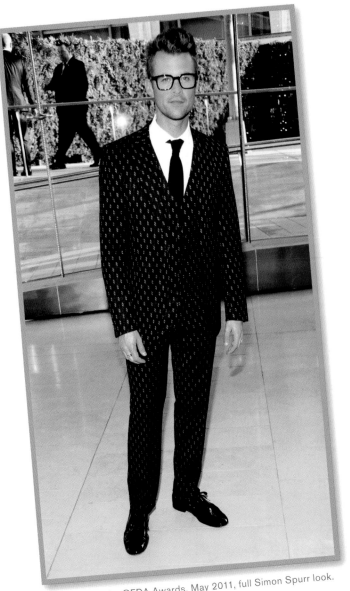

My first trip to the CFDA Awards, May 2011, full Simon Spurr look.

Ciao, Bella!

MY FIVE-SECOND GUIDE TO MILAN

Where to eat dinner: Da Giacomo, 6 Via Pascale Sottocorno
When you sit down for dinner at Da Giacomo, the waitstaff will
bring over a fresh slice of homemade pizza. But this is more
than a great restaurant (though it's that, too): Da Giacomo is *the*
hangout during Fashion Week—a place for models, designers, and
photographers to mingle and be merry.

Where to stay: Bulgari Hotel, 7/b Via Privata Fratelli Gabba
An extremely modern design—an aesthetic I savor—plus exceptional
service makes this the only place I'll stay in Milan. For breakfast, allow
me to recommend the pastry basket, which is full of croissants, *pains
au chocolat,* and baguettes. On a warm summer night, the courtyard
becomes one of Milan's best hotspots. You can't beat it.

Where to shop: Corso Como, 7d Via Alessio Di Tocqueville
A great shopping destination with an exceptional buy—if it's
happening in fashion, you can buy it here.

Where to eat lunch: Alla Cucina Delle Langhe, 6 Corso Como
Alla Cucina Delle Langhe is Tom Ford's favorite restaurant in
Milan, and with good reason. It's on the commercial promenade,
it's a place to see and be seen, and the food is delicious. From
squash blossoms to caprese salad and an exceptional antipasti
counter—dig in.

basement that we called "Store." It was basically a pretend Sears. This is
what life now felt like. Was I acting too quickly? What if I wound up back
in the garage?

So what. I would put the pieces of my business in place. And I would
reevaluate in a year. I was getting my name out there. I was saying, I'm

good at what I do. I'm proud of the work. It is a whole new beginning.

Suddenly I had one full-time administrative assistant and a part-time fashion assistant. We found an office; it was a one-bedroom apartment in a high-rise building made of glass. It was a gorgeous, 1,500-square-foot space of dark wood and new appliances and 15-foot ceilings with 180-degree views of the Hollywood Hills and downtown Los Angeles. I was in love. It made me happy to have somewhere to go every day. Even though my overhead was over my head.

I might have been a nervous wreck at times. But in Milan? For Fashion Week 2011? Well, there I felt like a star. I spent the afternoon with Anna Dello Russo from *Vogue* Japan—whom I'd dressed up as for Halloween! Inside her apartment, she told me, "I have enough fruit hats. I'm moving on to vegetables." And she did. She showed me a Carmen Miranda–style hat with all the elements of a salad on top. She is known for making music videos of herself dancing, and I walked into a shoot of her dancing to Lady Gaga's "The Edge of Glory." She asked if I wanted to make a video with her. (The answer was yes. I'm still waiting!)

I bore witness to the final fittings of the Dsquared² show. I went backstage to see Neil Barrett, who showed a punk, ska-influenced collection that I was obsessed with. Gary joined me, and it was his first Fashion Week. He was traveling in style, and so was I. I changed my clothing four times a day.

I had an audience with Donatella Versace. We'd met before, though I suspected she would not remember me. I prepared myself for this fact. Pierre Hardy, the French designer, introduced me. "This is Brad," he said.

"I know," Donatella said in that instantly recognizable deep-throated voice of hers. "I hear about Brad all of the time. Brad *this*. Brad *that*."

I loved that I was on her radar.

Back at home, every day was about finding new work. I was meeting with all of the Hollywood publicity agencies in town. These were general meetings where the celebrity publicists—the gatekeepers to the stars—could talk to me and get a sense of my style, away from what they knew from reality TV. This was my reality now, and the work followed. I dressed Abigail Spencer, a hot young actress from *Mad Men,* in Oscar de la Renta for the Comic-Con premiere of her film *Cowboys & Aliens.* I dressed the stunning Rashida Jones from *Parks and Recreation* for a premiere. *InStyle* asked me to curate a monthly page starting with September 2011. It's called "Brad's Buzz Board" and it's a roundup of the things that I am loving every month, as well as the celebrity red carpet looks I am obsessed with.

It was time to take stock of my life.

Cash flow was unpredictable, but my business was up and running. On a personal note, my ten-year anniversary with Gary was fast approaching, and he and I decided to throw a party. The plans started small, of course, but then escalated into a full-on catered backyard affair. We'd have to cover the pool to create a dance floor and we decided to bring in a DJ and professional lighting. Passed hors d'oeuvres gave way to a massive buffet. My mother and sister would fly in from Canada. I had a dozen friends flying in from New York. The guest list grew to some 150 people.

When I came out to my sister in high school, she was unfailingly supportive. What she didn't tell me then was the truth about her own fears, about what my homosexuality meant for *her* life. She'd looked forward to having a sister-in-law, to being an aunt. But talk to her today, and she will tell you that while Gary and I don't have kids, she doesn't feel she missed out on an ounce of life as my sister. Gary is her family as much as he is mine. It is not always like this for people out there, and I am grateful to have so much love in my life.

> "I wished my father and I could celebrate that together."

My father and I had been on very good terms up until recently. When I was in school, I was available to him. I'd go home and spend three days with my mom and then three days with him. In Alcoholics Anonymous,

making amends doesn't end with one conversation. It's called Living
the Amends. And I had been trying to be a better son. For his sixtieth
birthday, we went on a two-week bus tour of Italy. I'd send birthday cards,
Christmas cards, Thanksgiving cards. If there was a card for an occasion, I
sent one. But around the third season of *The Rachel Zoe Project,* I stopped
sending cards. I had more responsibility and was traveling and my job
was consuming my life. It had only gotten
worse since then.

> "Yes, I dressed Jessica
> Alba as Crystal Barbie."

My dad was angry at me. And he was
right. We'd drifted apart and it was my
fault. And sometimes I was short with him.
He'd say things to me like, "I don't understand what you do."

"You keep saying that," I'd say. "But there are three seasons of a
television show following me, showing exactly what I do. There's no clearer
explanation of what I do than that."

But my father shouldn't have to find out about my life from television.
I'd let my work put a wedge between us. And now I was trying to undo
it. I still am. My father said that I'd changed. That I'd become a different
person. What I wanted to say to him is this: I'm the exact same person
who came downstairs at age eleven with a comic book scarf tied around
his waist and wearing the jogging pants with the neon zippers. I wished
we could celebrate how far I'd come, from the day that I called him from
a street-corner pay phone in Toronto crying my eyes out, telling him I
needed to get sober, to where I am now, styling fashion shoots for major
magazines, filming my own TV show, and celebrating ten years in a
successful, stable relationship with a man who loves me. I wished my father
and I could celebrate that together. This was such an exciting time and
I didn't know how long it would last. Because if anyone knew how hard
it was for me to get here, and how unlikely this journey has been, it's my
father. After months of sorting out what our relationship would be we have

come to a mutual decision to let the past be the past and to move forward. We both want a relationship with each other that is lighter than it has been before. And in terms of all of the successes I've had this year, this could be the most important one. No matter how many miscommunications or misunderstandings you may have, your family is the most important thing and is worth fighting for.

In an odd way, through all of this, I was realizing how personal my work really is. Fashion was my savior when I was a kid. It gave me protection from the outside world. A way to announce what was in my heart when I couldn't find the words. And it would continue to be that for me. No more so than when I dressed Jessica Alba for the 2011 Met Ball.

The Costume Institute Gala, aka the Met Ball, sponsored by Anna Wintour and *Vogue* as a benefit for the Metropolitan Museum of Art's Costume Institute, is the fashion world's Oscars. It is the biggest night in fashion and an absolutely impossible ticket to get. Magazines and corporate sponsors pay $250,000 for a single table. Two hundred photographers line the red carpet. Inside, meanwhile, Gwyneth Paltrow mingles with Gisele Bündchen and Kristen

> "My work is meaningful to me because it's about more than playing dress-up. It's about making people feel at home in their own skin. It's about giving everyone their red carpet moment."

Stewart and Gwen Stefani and Jay-Z. It's one of the starriest rooms of the year. But someone once told me that the women's bathroom is where the real party goes down. It's the only place you can sneak a cigarette, plus you might see Mary-Kate and Ashley Olsen in ball gowns in a stall next to Coco Rocha.

I was dressing Jessica Alba for the 2011 Met Ball. Ralph Lauren invited her and of course offered to make her a custom gown for the night. This was thrilling but not without its challenges. A custom gown can be tricky. The way it looks sketched on the page isn't always how it turns out. The fit, the color—there are a lot of variables. The dress arrives, it's not what you think, and you have to scramble. It happens all the time. That wouldn't be an option here: She was Ralph's guest and she'd wear Ralph.

I struggled with an inspiration for the dress. Oh, did I mention that Jessica Alba would be seven months pregnant that night? This was the Met Ball. I didn't want her showing up in a muumuu. I wanted her to feel like she was dressed in something high-fashion. I wanted her to stand out in the crowd and get noticed.

I was flipping through a binder of recent Ralph Lauren gowns when I spotted a shape that would work for Jessica. And suddenly I had an emotionally charged flashback to my childhood. I was ten years old again and my favorite Barbie was Crystal Barbie. She had glass slippers and a sparkly, iridescent gown complete with layers of tulle. So much tulle! I remember losing one of Barbie's glass slippers, and even though it was really just a piece of see-through plastic with glitter in it, I cried. I thought, Without the right piece of footwear Barbie is just a shoeless tramp. But that dress!

I had a vision. Jessica Alba would go to the fashion world's Oscars in a sequined, custom-made Ralph Lauren gown with a platinum under-layer and beaded tulle. Yes, I dressed Jessica Alba as Crystal Barbie.

In a review of *The Rachel Zoe Project,* a writer for the *Los Angeles Times* suggested, "The idea that a person can get paid scads of money for telling someone else what to wear can also seem sort of, you know, wrong." But really, it was that reporter who got it wrong. I realized a stylist isn't a glorified personal shopper. We're being paid because we can see something a client can't. I'm being paid for the way my brain computes images and the way I see a puzzle coming together. My work is meaningful to me because it's about more than playing dress-up. It's about making people feel at home in their own skin. It's about giving everyone their red carpet moment.

When I saw Jessica Alba step out on the red carpet for the Met Ball, looking like a dream I once had, I cried. Not just for that night, but for this journey. Because I've proven everyone wrong. Because I've overcome so much. Because I am exactly where I am supposed to be.

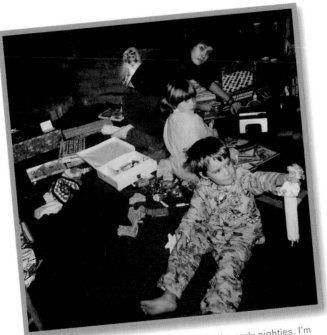

This was taken on a Christmas morning in the early eighties. I'm playing with my gift, Crystal Barbie, who also happened to be my inspiration for Jessica Alba's 2011 Met Ball look. My sister is in the background playing with her new train set, which I clearly had no interest in.

Epilogue:
You are the new black.

MY MOTHER ONCE TOLD me that she wanted to be a French teacher.

She wasn't a French teacher. No, for most of her adult life, she worked in her father's pharmacy. I remember my mom waking up every morning and putting on her uniform: the white cotton pants and the sensible shoes and the itchy standard-issue top. You could see the dissatisfaction and the frustration on her face.

I was twelve years old when she said to me, "Don't ever do something you don't love." She said it all the time. "Promise me," she said.

And that made such an impression on me.

It took me a long time to find out what I wanted to do. Yet when I look back on my life, it seems like it couldn't have been any other way. I was teased at school for dressing up like Madonna. Then I was in the basement making Fun Fur jackets with my mom. In high school, I styled my friend Tracy for the prom. All of these steps in my life—I didn't know what they were leading to, but everything, oddly, makes sense.

I feel like I'm doing exactly what I'm supposed to be doing. I'm lucky that I had people to encourage me along the way. Not everyone is so lucky. If your family isn't supportive, you have to make your own family. That's one of the joys of adult life. You can piece together your own support network.

If you are unhappy, I'm here to tell you: Make a change. Don't be afraid. What is the worst thing that could happen—you'll be unhappy in your new job? So what. You'll get another job.

A woman once said to me, "When you hear fear knocking on the door, most of the time when you answer it there's nothing there. It's just you holding yourself back."

I'm here to tell you: Let go.

The bullying I faced when I was younger helped me build a tougher skin. I spent all of that time at school pretending I didn't hear what the kids in the hallway were saying about me. Now, as an adult, I use those same skills to tune out the noise and focus on the work. Because it's the work I love.

At the time, I thought the bullies were breaking me down. But they only made me stronger. They helped me develop the courage to challenge myself. When I was drinking, I was only reflecting what I thought people saw in me—that I was this worthless kid from a small town. That I wasn't good at anything.

But that helps build a fire inside of you to propel you further. It's a great motivator: *I'll show you. I'll show you what I can do.*

What I want to say is this: If it can happen to me, it can happen to anybody. Maybe you think that is silly or cheesy. But it is the truth. Set the bar high for yourself. And grab it.

It takes a lot of hard work. I'm busier now than I've ever been, and

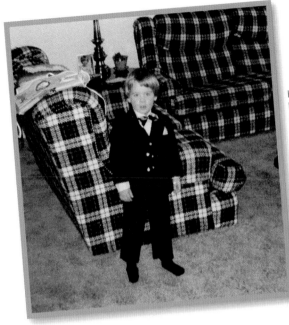

I apparently had a large stash of suits and bow ties from a young age. Here I am at around three dressed up yet again for a family occasion. You can see the beginnings of my signature look.

I'm my own boss. But it's a blessing. I'm glad I always wanted more for myself. And that I never stopped believing that I was good enough. My dream started small. I was good enough to go to community college. Then I thought, I'm good enough to get an internship. And then: I'm good enough to get an internship at *Vogue*.

Follow your passion. It's not about what your parents want you to be doing. I didn't go into fashion thinking I'd make money. When you take an entry-level position at a magazine, you can barely pay your rent. You cross your fingers and hope that ten years later you'll be an editor. But you do it because you love it. You have to do what you love. Believe in yourself. Believe that things are possible and they will happen.

Who knows what's next? But I know there is more out there. So many people come from this place of good enough. *This is my life. I'm happy here.* I've had those moments, but I've always pushed on. And I've never regretted reaching for more.

The other day during New York Fashion Week, I was sitting one bench behind Carine Roitfeld, the former editor in chief of French *Vogue.* She was in a full Givenchy look, on a Sunday morning at the Victoria Beckham show, and I was in awe. Sometimes I think being an outsider is just as exciting as being an insider. Because you get to fantasize about what it would be like to be at a table somewhere having tea with her.

That's part of what makes me get out of bed every day and want to do this job. It makes me want to do good work. To get to the next marker. To the next milestone.

I try not to look back, but sometimes I do. And I see myself a decade ago, at a crossroads, still using and unable to sleep, staring at myself in the mirror and thinking my life was empty. Thinking this was the end for me. But here I am: I own my own business. I travel to Milan for Fashion Week. And Donatella Versace knows my name. If that isn't proof that anything can happen, I don't know what is.

I was born to be Brad.

"Ignore the bullies and find out where your true passion lies, and when you're ready, make it happen."

Acknowledgments

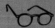

I cannot thank Mickey Rapkin enough for all of his hard work and dedication. He had enthusiasm for this book from the moment I told him I had the idea to the moment we submitted the final draft. Thank you! I feel so lucky to have had the chance to work on this with you!

To Penelope and Jasper for reminding me that no matter how stressful things are, all that matters is love.

To my dad for his love and support.

To Eric Kranzler, Chris Huvane, and Darin Friedman—I appreciate everything you do for me more than you can imagine.

To Tracy Doyle, Danielle Nachmani, Annebet Duvall, and Trish Lahde for always being there for me through thick and thin.

To my assistants, Lindsay Myers and Thomas Carter

Phillips, who are a joy to see every day. They work hard and laugh hard. I couldn't do anything without you and am grateful to have you in my life.

To John and Felicia Janetti, Maria, Adam, and Sarah and Emily Abeshouse for accepting me into your family with open arms.

To Jessica Alba for taking a chance on me! I will always be grateful to you. It is an absolute pleasure working with you.

To *InStyle* magazine for giving me my first major fashion shoot. Thank you for your trust in my abilities.

To Joe Zee for your friendship and support right from the beginning.

To Prabal Gurung—thank you for your wisdom and great advice. It has been invaluable.

To Amy Bendell, Lisa Sharkey, Farley Chase, Carrie Kania, Andrea Rosen, Cal Morgan, Alberto Rojas, Kevin Callahan, Lorie Pagnozzi, Joyce Wong and Renato Stanisic—thank you for your guidance and enthusiasm through this process.

To Andy Cohen, Ryan Flynn, Shari Levine, and Frances Berwick at Bravo—I feel so blessed to be part of the Bravo family.

To Jen O'Connell, Nick Emmerson, and Stephanie Chambers at Shed Media—I cannot thank you enough for your hard work and belief in the show.

To Yu Tsai—thanks for pulling the shoot together for me and giving me a gorgeous book cover.

To Ron F. for helping me build a spiritual foundation.

To Jhoni Marchinko and Sara Switzer—thank you for helping me get my internship at *Vogue*. You made my dream come true.

To Candie Weitz, everything changed for me the night you took me to the Chanel Fine Jewelry dinner. I cannot thank you enough for your kindness and your friendship.

To Diane Lackie for your love and encouragement.

To Tom and Catherine Millar—I am so grateful to you both for making my childhood a magical one. My years in the Scugog Choral Society and the Millarlights are deeply cherished.